Iron Body
Workout like the Gods, Goddesses of Olympus

Frank Marchante

Gras Publishing, Miami, Florida

Iron Body-Workout like the Gods, Goddesses of Olympus

© 2023 by Frank Marchante

Published by Gras Publishing Company.
Miami, Florida

Copyright © 2023 by Frank Marchante

Library of Congress Control Number: 2022920035
Marchante, Frank
Iron body-Workout like the gods, goddesses of Olympus
2/10/2023
Pages 338
ISBN 978-0-97790-40-0-6

Front cover photo 1 by:
Freepick.com user Drobotdean

Front cover photo 2 by:
Unsplash.com user Darren Lawrence

Back cover photo by:
Pixabay.com user Frabicio Macedo

This book is printed in Acid free paper.
Printed in the United States of America

1. Bodybuilding. 2. Women's Fitness. 3. Cardiovascular fitness.
4. Exercise hand book manual. 5. Weight loss. 6. Health & Fitness.
7. Exercise. 8. Aerobics. 9. Strength Training. 10. Diet & Nutrition.

Dedication

This book has countless roots. Before anything else, I'd like to thank God for the infinite blessings, inspiration, and energy. Thanks to my parents, whose first response was always, "How can we help?" to Mom and Dad, all that I owe to you. Mom, I can feel your presence with me every day, and you are my guardian angel. My father was an extraordinary man, my teacher and a friend. I wouldn't be the man I'm today if it weren't for the parents I had. Thank you once again.

My sister, I love my sister, Babie, who has always been there. To my wonderful children, Monica, Michelle, and Franky, I love you all more than anything. My wife, Gilda, for always been there. This book is also dedicated to my granddaughters Sofia, Ali, Ayla, and my grandson Georgie.

I also want to dedicate this book to all the people who have inspired me throughout all of my years. Especially growing up, Charles Atlas was my first encounter with a muscular body (the skinny guy at the beach in the comic book). I was also fascinated as a young boy by Johnny Weissmuller playing Tarzan in the movies.

My second glimpse of a strong bodybuilding icon was of Steve Reeves playing Hercules on the movie screen. This was the moment when I said to myself, "I want to be in shape." At 12 years old, Steve Reeves in the Hercules movie was responsible for me starting to exercise. Then, Bruce Lee and Chuck Norris, a karate champion, inspired me to continue my self-defense training.

A particular thanks to Denie, a superb-charismatic famous author, photographer, and publisher who has now become a family friend and has provided me with a wealth of ideas and pointers, including many of his well-known images. The late Robert Kennedy, Musclemag-Reps publisher-owner, the late Joe Weider, co-founded the International Federation of Bodybuilders (IFBB). Muscle Builder-Flex, Muscle Power-Mr. America owner-publisher, also Dan Lurie, founding father of Bodybuilding WBBG (world record holder for amazing feats of strength)-Muscle Training Illustrated publisher, made history in 1984 by arm wrestling U.S. president Ronald Reagan in the Oval office.

Peary and Mabel Rader, founders and publishers of Iron Man Magazine; Bob Hoffman, founder of the York Barbell Company; and magazines such as Muscular Development and Strength & Health, publisher.

My thanks to Sergio Oliva, my teenage hero and inspiration. If he could make it, I could too. Sergio became my friend. Little did I know at the time that his body was one in a million. Not only did he have physical perfection, but he became one of the greatest bodybuilders ever. A man who placed honesty, rather than commercialism, first.

Arthur Jones, an incredibly knowledgeable man, developed HIT (the High Intensity Training), the founder of Nautilus equipment, Mike Mentzer (developed the Heavy Duty System), and Vince Gironda (the guru of bodybuilding). I became a follower of these three men's training concepts.

I also want to mention the champions I grew up with, admired, looked after, and learned from all of them. Anibal Lopez, The late Dave Draper (The blond bomber), Frank Zane, the late Franco Columbo, Arnold Schwarzenegger, Lou Ferrigno, Casey Viator ("The youngest ever Mr. America at age 19"), Ed Corney, Christ Dickerson, Dennis Tinerino, Dorian Yates, John Grimek, Jay Cutler, Ray Mentzer, Reg Park, Freddy Ortiz, Harold Poole, Don Horworth, Mike Mentzer, the late Serge Nubret-(The Black Panther),Tom Platz, and many other champions who inspired me. I learned from them. I felt like I knew them all.

To my students, you know who you are, and I'm speaking directly to each of you. You all make my life such a joy and an unforgettable experience. Most of all, my gratitude goes to each and every student that has graced my path. To all these individuals, and many others who have helped me along the way, I'm deeply indebted. Without them, this book could not have been possible. I'm grateful and want to thank them all.

I hope this book helps people to achieve the bodies of their dreams, maintain their general health, and obtain strength and mobility for a lifetime of living!

Acknowledgements

I want to thank Michelle, my daughter, for her support, input, insight, and creativity. I could not have completed this book without her help. I also want to thank my wife, Gilda, for her patience and for always being there.

My son Franky, who has helped me with many of his gym photos,

Again, I would like to thank all those people, champions, writers, Muscle Magazine Publishers, and photographers, that inspired me to train my whole life.

I would also like to thank Denie, the legendary- mythical writer-editor-photographer, gym owner and commercial consultant in the health and fitness industry, and all the photographers, many of whom are named on the credit page at the back of the book.

I would like to recognize those who have inspired me, either directly or indirectly.

I have not attempted to cite all authorities and sources in the preparation of this book, like departments of the government, periodicals, websites, libraries, institutions, and many individuals.

I sincerely thank all these people.

Thanks to all of you!

Warning-Disclaimer

The materials presented in this book are for "informational and entertainment purposes only." Before participating in any physical activity, you should consult your physician and ask for a complete exam, including a stress test. Especially if you have never exercised, are pregnant, or suffer from any kind of illness. As with all exercise and dietary programs, you should get your doctor's approval before beginning, and agree to be of legal age and use the information responsibly.

The exercise and dietary programs in this book are not intended as a substitute for any exercise or dietary regimen that may have been prescribed by your doctor.

You should be aware that if you follow any of the advice included in this book, you are doing so entirely at your own risk, which includes any past, present, or future physical, medical, or psychological pain or injury whatsoever that you may incur or receive.

The author and publisher should bear no liability or responsibility to any person or entity for any loss or damage caused, or alleged to be caused, directly or indirectly by the information in this book.

This book contains the author's personal opinions.

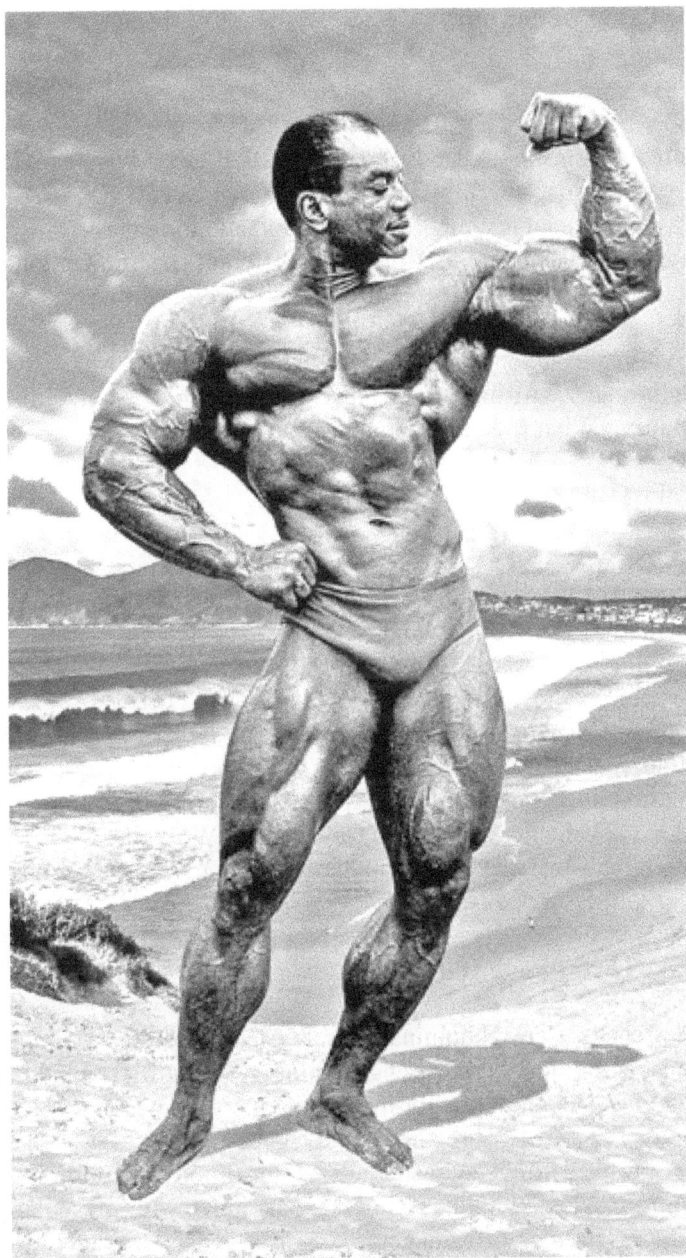

Sergio Oliva Mr. Olympia- Mr.Olympus- Mr.Universe
Photo Courtesy of Wayne Galash

A Table of content

Part Four- page 159

Miscellaneous excellent exercises -Tire Exercises
Medicine Ball-Hammer workout
Train like a Fighter-Jumping Rope for a Fighter body
Sprint Training
Free Exercise Routine Woman -Woman Basic Routines
Intermediate/advance routine-Advance woman Routine workout.
Cardio Explanation
Men Beginners Workout-Intermediate/Advance routine
Abdomen-Crunches-Vacuum
Add ¼ to ½ inches to your arms-Secret-Muscle Mass-Bulking/Mass-
Mass training-Working out/cardio-Injury-What to Wear.

Part Five-page 229

Old School Training to gain a massive 25 pounds of muscle
Eating for huge massive bulk-Fiver/Foods for Weight Loss-Ideas to
Cut Calories- Avoid Gaining Weight -Yo-yo diet theory-On the Go-
Sugar-Muscle burn more calories than fat-Men Health -Testosterone -
Theories why we age, lose ability, and die.
GH -Main systems of the human body -Where's the beef? Glutes
Sleek, strong, sexy-Ass most women want a first-class ass -Ass
Sexy Glutes -Waist –Thigh Trimming
Woman's Core Muscles-Spot Reducing-The truth how to lose weight
Sprints-Exercises that thicken the waist should be avoided
What to Eat to Lose Belly Fat-Nutrition rules.

Part Six-page 289

Cellulite-Pregnant
Muscle burns more calories than fat- Calorie- Fast foods
Sample of Muscle weight gain Diets lose weight samples
Lose fat –Beer-Normal aging-Testosterone-Mature Bodybuilding-The
Mature Weight Gainer-Aspirin - The Wonder Drug-Steroids-
Alzheimer's disease-Common training injuries-Conclusion-Keep a
log-Terminologies worth knowing-About the Author-Photo Credit
Media related –Books Periodicals / websites-Reviews.

Introduction

You are never too old or too out of shape to get into better shape! It's realistic to see a transformation in four weeks. With these kick-ass workout programs, you will be shedding fat like never before.

You have in your possession the key to unlocking the body of your dreams. No crap, just the important and essential strategies with the tools to help you get the body of your dream. This book is going to unlock your best body in record time. These workouts will make you sleek, crazy sexy, and in top shape. I have chosen exercises that target your entire body with different kinds of methods and equipment, including free calisthenics exercises.

If you are a woman, these mind-boggling workouts will give you a lean and sexy look, a body that will fit into an attractive butt-twitcher Brazilian bikini, and if trying on your favorite skirt is causing you distress because of the condition of your thighs, you can correct that. If you want the perfect bikini body, lean and with tight curves in all the right places, and if you want it fast, this book is for you.

It's true that genetics plays a large part in how much you can reshape this area of your body, but I promise you, you can make a transformation with exercises. The question always comes out. Are women working out going to get bulky? The struggle for women to achieve and maintain a lean, defined, strong body is doubly harder than it is for men.

Exercise helps men and women in different ways. Most women will achieve a lean and toned body. Numerous women believe that if they lift weights, they're going to bulk up. Not true. The result is a nice shape and a sexy body.

The exercises in this book will help you tone and develop these important muscles, and consider the aesthetic benefits you'll see, sleeker, shapelier hips and trimmer thighs, an incredible bonus.

This also applies to men with skinny legs. If you are a guy, the following workouts will have you in shape like nothing ever before.

Total body transformation. Friends will be asking you for your secret! What's been stopping you from having the body of your dreams? It's about time you went out and got that sexy, attractive, strong, and in shape body. There's a right way and a wrong way to get in shape. If you've been exercising with nothing to show for it, this book is for you.

Do you have experience in any of these situations? Going to the gym or exercising every month without seeing any progress? Doing cardio for hours with no significant loss in weight loss? Quitting exercising out of frustration?

Stop doing the same exercises that haven't given you any results; try my way of acquiring a lean and ripped body. What do you have to lose? If you receive your information from a commercial magazine, keep in mind that their primary existence is to sell products. I'm not saying supplements are not good; some are incredibly good. In my younger years, I tried some of them, and got really good results with some of them. Just do your homework and learn.

You have the key and the guide to that body in your hands. Is it going to be easy? No, this book will not give you abs, but this book is your road map to an incredibly attractive body, but you have to implement and do the workouts, any of them.

You are not going to get a sexy, in-shape, strong muscle body by only reading this book. You must do any of the workouts listed in this book.

Here you will also find nutrition advice that'll kick fad diets goodbye. You'll eat awesome food and enjoy your dinner time without being restricted or going hungry. I'll recommend a straightforward "eat clean" approach, with no strange gimmicks, wacky diets, or calorie counting. In this book, I'm addressing men and women as him/her or you.

You will find in this book complete workout descriptions, information on a variety of options for workouts like cardio training, running, jogging, free calisthenics, isometric workouts, spring/cable training, bands, Power Twist, weight training, mass building, ass shaping, fighter workouts, including proper warm-up, cool-down, and injury prevention techniques, the proper way to eat, and much more.

If you picked this book with the hope of getting new ideas to enhance your workouts, you have made a good choice. The format of this book is simple. I have dedicated my entire life to instructing people. I have learned by reading, training, listening, and observing experts the proper way of working out for over 50 years, and it is from their wealth of experience that I present this book. This book is not a guarantee of a Mr. America or Ms. Physique.

Like all advice to you, you should take my advice just like any other advice. Keep in mind that I've gathered my judgment not only through personal trial and error but also by exchanging training ideas with several of the most well-known bodybuilding champions and prominent trainers in the world.

For years, I remember reading anything I could get my hands on about bodybuilding, physical culture, physical training, and medical articles and books. I felt it was necessary to address certain medical topics in this work.

As a teenager, I remember eagerly anticipating the arrival of the muscle magazine on the newsstand each month, buying all of them, and learning from the writers and champions on the subject. I read those articles carefully and many times, two or three times. This is what motivated me to meet some champions and looked for Sergio Oliva. I looked all over and could not find his book. This was the way Sergio Oliva the Myth book was born. He did not have one, so I wrote one.

As a professor in the four largest school districts in the USA for 30 years, I guided many young men to make it to the football team. Some went on to win local bodybuilding contests, including my son Franky.

I have read hundreds of articles and probably hundreds of books in my 50 years of involvement in health, training, and learning, not only in exercise and training but also in medicine, major diseases, and rehabilitation.

Some medical issues included in this book I felt were critical to providing some specific information. Occasionally, after leaving the doctor's office, friends and family members call me to discuss the results or ask me to review the drug prescription, my thoughts on specific medications, their lab results, or discuss the CAT Scam or MRI results.

I'm not a bodybuilder or fighting champion, not a doctor or a nurse, but I bet you I know what I'm writing about.

If you are a woman, you are probably thinking, what does this author know about feminine culture? A short answer is, I've been married for over 36 years, have two grown daughters, and three teenage girl grandkids. As a professor for 30 years, I had thousands of students. Half of those were girls. I heard about the complaint they made, many times I served as a counselor. Apart from reading medical materials, I have also spoken to many bodybuilders' female champions and health writers and publishers.

You are reading this book because you don't want to read a science degree book; you are reading it because you want to get into awesome shape fast. You are probably thinking about next year's swimsuit, or tight jeans, or how to look nice and in shape in your men's suit. Findings show that exercise reduces your risk of many serious ailments, including heart disease, stroke, colon cancer, and diabetes, helping you obtain strong bones, muscles, and joints, and, in many cases, easing arthritis pain. It's also a great way to relieve stress.

These days, we have to get through the day, probably with no physical exertion at all. What do we do in the evening? Slouch onto the couch and watch TV. How many of you sit for long hours all day long?

You must exercise to keep in shape. Moreover, if you're trying to lose weight, working out is a must.

No matter if it's a brisk walk around the block, cardio, or weight training session at the gym, your body uses body fat to provide the energy needed to complete that activity. Remember, exercise builds muscle and helps you burn calories even when you're at rest.

According to the American College of Sports Medicine, you should do at least 30 minutes of moderate exercise three or four days a week for adults to stay healthy. Training became a passion, and I valued sharing it with people.

However, sitting down and putting everything in writing was not something easy to do.

When I'm talking to people, the age factor always comes up. Again, I'll be honest with you. I never think about aging. When I was in my 40's, I was in much better shape than people 20 years younger. I've used these concepts throughout my training years and remained injury free. I still love to exercise. The thought of exercising still excites me. Of course, I don't work-out as hard as I used to during my younger years and I don't go to my maximum.

Sergio Oliva the Myth thought, like I also think, that it was an error to copy someone else's training because everyone has singular needs and potentials. That's why I'm combining in this book different and general techniques so each individual can choose the one best appropriate for themselves.

Rather than confusing you with many never-ending details and exercises like "There is no tomorrow, "To leave your head spinning, I present the information simply and to the point. If you want to learn more about science, you will be reading another kind of book.

"The journey of a thousand miles begins with one step"
Lao Tzu's

Shock-Body Transformation

I've been exercising, practicing boxing, Kung Fu, and lifting weights in some form or another since 12 years old. In my teenage years, I became passionate about body building and fitness. I bought and read every fitness and muscle magazine available at the time. I have spent a lot of years, money, and effort over the last 50 years. I have learned what really works and what doesn't when it comes to fitness. Do I know everything? No, of course not. Nobody knows everything.

But I can teach you techniques that took me years of trial and error to learn.

Today, I still enjoy the many benefits of bodybuilding and different approaches to training, of course, with less intensity. I never wanted to be big, with veins pumping out, just lean, trim, and agile. Not everyone is born with the genetics to be a champion or to be big and strong.

I also believe that not everyone can be a top champion; you need to have the perfect genes, workout extremely hard, make immense sacrifices, and have a lot of determination. It's not an easy task!

It is verified that weight training helps develop muscle mass and strengthens your bones. Bodybuilding gives you a feeling of vitality and, at the same time, makes your muscles look toned and strong, improves posture, and makes you look really good in a swim suit or a jean, no matter if you are a woman or a man, giving you an attractive and sexy body. You don't need to go to a gym or buy expensive equipment. You could train in your home with a set of free weights and a bench; your own body can be your gym; that's all you need.

If you want a shocking body transformation, you must do a powerful explosion of intense exercises. My training method, which I have been practicing for many years, works great for me and for almost everybody who has tried it. As you progress, it is a must to do the same number of circuits in less time.

These circuits are challenging. Make sure they don't interfere with your weight-training progress.

The purpose of these circuits is to increase your conditioning, athleticism, mobility, and burn body fat. Many experts believe, including me, that walking (training) in the morning before you eat leads to faster fat loss. You don't have to do strenuous cardio in a fasted state; a brisk walk or a small bicycle ride is fine. Take a small coffee before your **real** workout. Working with weight resistance is the ultimate body training!

This book will give you short routines and circuits that you can do anywhere, anytime.

Set small goals.

My process is simple, and it's been working for me since I was a teenager. I set a small goal, and then when I archive that goal, I make another small goal, then another, and another. Reaching my total or big goal at the end is easier because it's easier to archive small goals one at a time than go for a big, almost impossible to reach goal.

I believe morning cardio workouts can improve digestion, decrease body weight and fat, and improve sleep quality, among many other benefits.

Do I have all the answers? No, nobody has all the answers, but in over 50 years, I have met and discussed many issues from training to diets with many champions, like Mr. America, Mr. Universe, and martial arts experts. For example, the great champion Sergio Oliva, winner of over 50 titles including Mr. America, Mr. Universe, Mr. World, Mr. Olympia, Mr. Olympus, and many others.

"Honesty is the first chapter in the book of wisdom"
Thomas Jefferson

Get a Physical

The first thing you should do before starting any exercise program is to have your doctor gives you a check-up. A complete physical, including a stress test, is a good idea, and when you get a clean bill of health from your physician, start slowly. Take your time. It took you years to get out of shape, so don't try to get in shape in a hurry.

The American Heart Association recommends a minimum of two and a half hours a week of moderate exercise.

Heart attack warning symptoms are:

Chest pain-pressure   Fainting-fatigue
Dizziness   Stomach pains
Weakness   Shortness of breath
 Nausea   Sweating

If you have any of these problems, please consult your doctor before training.

High blood pressure   Obesity
History of heart disease   Sedentary life
High cholesterol

If at any time you feel bad, stop right away! Call your doctor and have him look into the problem.

Understand your past:

Most importantly, make sure you know about your family.
Did anyone in your family die under the age of fifty?
Did anyone have a heart attack?
Does someone in your family have diabetes, high cholesterol, high blood pressure, or high triglycerides?
Do you have a waist measurement greater than 35 inches?
If you smoke, stop. This is the most important thing you can do for those around you.

HISTORY

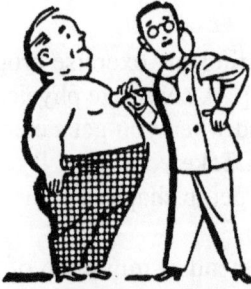

Our predecessor needed to walk and work all of the time. Alan Calvert invented the plate-loading barbell around the turn of the century. The society in which we live is an inactive society. Your co-worker at the office is 20 feet from your desk; you e-mail him/her instead of walking there to talk. Americans are overweight and out of shape. Think about it. When was the last time you walked to the grocery store? When was the last time you took a walk in the park after dinner? I have deduced your response.

A Complete Fitness Routine

A complete fitness routine should focus on endurance, strength, flexibility, and balance. Stick to my guidance of rotating the exercises of doing weights, sprinting, free exercising, and the other training disciplines I mention in other parts of this book.

You will be shocked at the way your body is going to feel and look in a matter of months. You are in for a surprise. But you have to work at it.

Balance should be very important to everybody, including athletes. Generally, training routines focus on the visible muscles. The work outs described in this book will increase your power, coordination, and balance and should be a factor in everyone's training.

Muscle memory

I'm familiar myself, and any person who has lifted weights, on and off, is familiar with the well-known concept of muscle memory. Muscle memory is the concept that it is much easier to go back to your old shape than those just beginning to get in shape.

Generic

Genes are the fundamental physical unit of heredity. Your genetics completely regulate your natural growth. Some of us are born with narrow shoulders, while others have wide clavicles, thick wrists, and a powerful response to training. A bigger bone structure comes with a bigger muscle. Heredity, also called inheritance or biological inheritance, is the transmission of traits from parents to their offspring; you inherited half of your genes from your mother. You inherited half of your genes from your father. Genes are a kind of code.

Your genes determine your size, the strength of your body, and even how healthy you are. You have no control over the situation. If you have narrow shoulders, you can compensate by doing a lot of shoulder exercises. If you are a woman with skinny legs, you can improve by doing a lot of leg exercises.

But you can only improve to a point because of your genetics. Your genetic heritage is responsible for inherited fat (adipose cells). When you see men with ripped and bulking muscles and women with beautiful bodies, you can tell they have better genetics than the rest of us. You can influence roughly half of how young, strong, and trim you are, according to some experts; the other half is dictated by your genes. We must try our best with the genes we inherit.

Muscle

A muscle has three levels of strength: positive (raising), static (holding), and negative (lowering). Muscles are groups of tissues that cross joints in the body. When they contract, they produce movements that shorten the distance between the joints.

Lower Body Muscles

The gastrocnemius, soleus, and calf, upper legs, the hamstring group, and the quadriceps, the front of the legs.

Upper body muscles

The chest pectoralis major/minor, the muscles in the back the latissimus dorsi (lats), the trapezius, and the muscles of the shoulders (the deltoids)

Biceps

The two main muscles in your upper arms are the biceps in front and the triceps in back. They are opposing muscle functions. The biceps brachii, known as the biceps, is a double-headed muscle that runs from the shoulder to the elbow. They are involved in lifting and pulling with the arms.

Triceps

The triceps The brachii, also known as the triceps, are a group of three muscles located at the back of your arms. These muscles run between your shoulder and elbows. Their function is to strengthen your arms and stabilize your shoulders.

Forearm

There are three muscles in the deep anterior forearm: flexor digitorum profundus, flexor pollicis longus, and pronator quadratus. There are five in the posterior forearm: the supinator, abductor pollicis longus, extensor pollicis brevis, extensor pollicis longus, and extensor indicis.

Core

These muscles play an important role in everyday activities like walking, bending over to pick up a box, and most importantly, keeping you upright. The rectus abdominis, also known as the six-pack, is located in front of the torso; the transverse abdominis is located on each side of the naval; the internal and external oblique extend diagonally from the ribs to the pelvis; and the multifidus and spinal erector are located along the spine from head to pelvis.

Ligaments and tendons

Tendons connect muscles to bone, and ligaments attach bones to bones. Proper warm-up is a must to keep them injury-free.

Joints

The human body contains more than a hundred joints, 143 to be exact. Strong, flexible joints are essential for almost every activity of daily living. Unfortunately, joint problems are one of the leading causes of disability in the United States and around the world.

Cartilage

They are considered the body's shock absorbers. Their primary function is to keep bones from rubbing against each other while moving.

Skeletal muscle

Skeletal muscle mainly attaches to the skeletal system via tendons to maintain posture and control movement. The first and most apparent function of the skeletal system is to provide a framework for the body

Obesity

Fat is not your enemy. Fat does not make you fat. Your body needs fat because healthy fat is an essential source of good cholesterol. Not all cholesterol is bad.

Cholesterol

The two types of cholesterol are LDL cholesterol, which is bad, and HDL, which is good.
LDL (bad) cholesterol narrows the arteries and increases the risk of heart attack and stroke.
At a healthy level, HDL (good) cholesterol may protect against heart attack and stroke. The National Cancer Institute states that high cholesterol raises the risk of breast cancer by 25 percent.

Triglycerides

Triglycerides are the most common type of fat in the body. A high triglyceride level combined with high LDL (bad) cholesterol or low HDL (good) cholesterol is linked to fatty buildups within the artery walls, which increases the risk of heart attack and stroke.

Metabolism

Scientists use it to describe the chemical processes in the body, especially those that involve nutrients.

The American Diabetes Association

Points out that people with diabetes have an increased risk of cardiovascular events like heart attacks and strokes.

Blood pressure

When your heart contracts, pressure is created. This is called the systole, and when the heat relaxes, the pressure is called diastole. The American Heart Association recommends, as of 2022, less than 120 mmHg and less than 80 mmHg-120/80 mmHg.

Heart

During a workout, blood pressure and heart rate rise, and the heart pumps a greater volume of blood than when we are at rest. Monitor your heart rate, you should learn how to find your resting heart rate.

Use this simple formula:
220-your age = then multiply the MHR by certain percentages to determine the right heart rate "zones" to exercise in:

50 to 70 percent (MHR x.5 to.7) for an easy workout.
Moderate workout, 70 to 85 percent (MHR x.7 to.85) for a moderate
Aim for 85 to 95 percent (MHR x.85 to.95) for an intense workout.

"Take care of your body. It's the only place you have to live"
Jim Rohn

What does it mean?

Aerobic means requiring free oxygen to meet the energy needs through exercise by way of aerobic. That indicates that walking, running, swimming, cycling, dancing, and hiking are all aerobic.

In a study done by researchers at the University of British Columbia, it was learned that consistent aerobic exercise increased the size of the hippocampus, the part of the brain involved in both verbal memory and learning.

In the same research, the same outcomes were not seen in those who only executed balance exercises, resistance training, and muscle toning exercises.

Similar experimental conclusions were repeated during a similar study that took place at the University of Illinois at the Urbana-Champaign campus.

This study indicated that when individuals between the ages of 55 and 80 frequently did a walking routine for a year, the hippocampus, which normally loses mass as we age, increased in size.

People who exercise aerobically are more likely to experience better sleep, have a better mood, and, at the same time, their anxiety and stress levels are reduced.

Teeth

I have seen many books dedicated to health and achieving a nice, strong, trim, attractive body, but they don't mention how important it is to have nice teeth. That's why I'm mentioning the teeth here. Your teeth are one of the strongest parts of your body. Every time we smile, frown, talk, or eat, we use our mouths and teeth. The mouth is essential for speech. Together with the lips, tongue, and teeth, it helps form words. The human teeth function by breaking down food by cutting and crushing them to prepare them for swallowing and digesting.

According to the Academy of General Dentistry, more than 90 percent of diseases that produce oral signs and symptoms will be prevented by brushing your teeth and keeping them healthy. This will prevent many health issues. Gum disease can increase your risk of heart disease.

It includes:
Strokes   Diabetes mellitus
Heart disease   Kidney issues
Lung infections

Your teeth help you keep your jaw bone strong. They are connected to your gums, and the gums are connected to your jawbone, so if you lose some teeth, they will misalign your jaw. People notice teeth as the first thing when they meet and interact with a person; they make assumptions right away based on your teeth. People with healthy, nice, clean teeth are viewed as attractive and successful people.

You should brush your teeth at least 3 times a day, and every time you brush your teeth scrap or brush your tongue, the tongue is a host of bacteria and will cause bad breath. You should also floss. Every day or depending on your hearth teeth.

Periodontal disease Risk:
Family history- genetics-hormonal changes-not brushing or flossing

Hair

Again, like I said in the tooth section, I have seen many books dedicated to health and achieving a nice, strong, trim, attractive body, but they don't mention anything about hair, or being bold. That's why I'm mentioning it here.

Hair is mostly made up of a protein called keratin.It grows from follicles in the dermis. Hair loss makes men and women look old and can negatively impact their overall attractiveness. In fact, hair in general can have an impact on people's perceptions of a man's or woman's age.

In men, hair loss is the number one physical trait that people perceive to age a man. It can even add up to eight years.

According to clinical research, hair that is grey comes in second and can add up to seven years.

Male pattern baldness is a hereditary hair loss condition most likely passed on by the **father's side of the family.**

There are numerous reasons why women might experience hair loss. Anything from medical conditions to hormonal changes to stress may be the reason.

The most common type of hair loss in men and women is androgenetic alopecia, or baldness or hair loss caused by genetics or family history.

Hereditary hair loss with age is the most common cause of baldness.

Hair loss is typically related to one or more of the following factors:

- **Family history (heredity).** The most common cause of hair loss is hereditary.

- **Hormonal changes and medical conditions** like pregnancy, childbirth, menopause, and thyroid problems.

- **Medications and supplements** can be a side effect of certain drugs.

- **Stress** thinning of hair after several months of stress.

Hair care tips

Wash your hair regularly with the use of chemical-free shampoos.

Blow drying-excessive heat can damage your hair scalp

Dry your hair naturally by air drying or using a towel.

Don't wash your hair frequently; wash it every 3–4 days.

Eat healthy; your hair is made of protein and amino acids.

Drink water. Internal and external hydration is key to healthy hair.

Hair don'ts

Hot showers strip off natural oil from your scalp, leaving it dry.

Stress can cause hair to fall out. Try to reduce stress.

Caps-Sun rays–use hats to protect the hair. The sun removes moisture from the hair, making it dry and brittle.

Swimming pool-protect your hair from chlorinated water with a cap.

A shaved head-a symbol of aggression and toughness

Greek soldiers during the reign of Alexander the Great were ordered to shave their heads as a defensive measure, so the enemy during hand-to-hand battle could not grab their hair.

A shaved head has become a symbol of aggression and toughness.

About a hundred years ago, the only people you saw with shaved heads were the prisoners trying to control lice in jail.

Over the years, other groups have adopted the bald look, like the skinheads, neo-Nazis, and other groups, to make a rebellious statement.

Can a bald man look more attractive? People perceive bald men as more intelligent and dominant than men with a full head of hair.

Bald men stand out from the crowd; they look stronger and more powerful than an average man. Shaved heads have their disadvantages. These men were rated as less attractive and at least four years older than guys with a full head of hair.

Many of the biggest tough guys in Hollywood keep shaved heads, like Bruce Willis, The Rock, and many others. Many of the biggest tough guys in Hollywood keep shaved heads, like Bruce Willis, The Rock, and many others.

Albert Mannes from the University of Pennsylvania's Wharton School of Business did a research paper titled "Shorn Scalp and Perceptions of Male Dominance." It was published in the journal Social Psychological and Personality Science, and he did three experiments.

1-Are men with shaved heads perceived as more dominant?

The shaved men topped the ratings for how powerful and influential they looked.

2-Does a bald man increase a man's perception of strength?

The men with shaved heads not only came across as more dominant, but also an inch taller and 13% stronger.

3-Thinning hair, shaved head or full hair?

The men with shaved heads were rated highest in dominance, masculinity, and strength. The guys with a full head of hair scored higher for attractiveness than the bald men.

Only you can decide if you want to shave all of your hair. You have to keep in mind the shape of your head, ears, and body size when wearing this. My son has been shaving his head since he was fourteen years old, and he looks great.

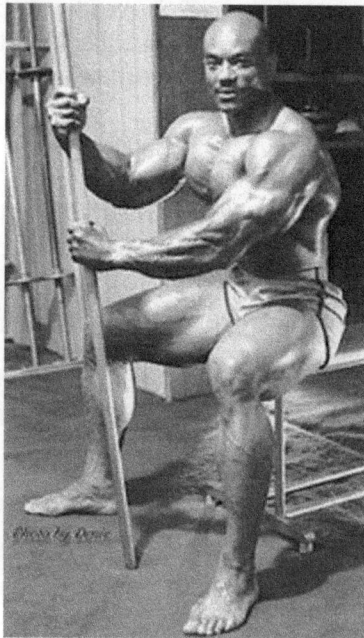

Photo by Denie

Tan

Everybody wants to have a tan. A tan makes a man or woman look healthy, sexy, in shape, and more attractive.

Bodybuilders' champions get a tan to look more impressive on the day of the competition. Black champions like the amazing Robby Robinson, the Black Prince, and the mindboggling Sergio Oliva, the Myth, both claim they use it to get a tan because it makes their muscles lose water and look muscular and cut.

Be careful with tanning beds. According to the American Academy of Dermatology association, just one tanning bed session increases a person's chances of developing:

Melanoma by 20%
Squamous cell carcinoma by 67%

Tips:

Avoid excessive time in the sun in one session. It is better to tan at shorter intervals. Avoid the sun from 10.00 a.m. until 2.00 p.m., when UV rays are strongest.

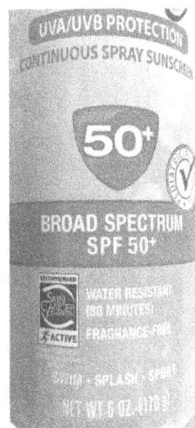

The American Academy of dermatology says a tan is not a sign of health. It's a sign that you have damaged your skin. Regularly apply a broad spectrum sunscreen of at least SPF 30. Make sure to re-apply after swimming. Wear a hat and sunglasses with 99/100% UVA and UVB protection to protect the scalp and eyes.

Keep in mind that sand, snow, and water all reflect the sun's rays, and sometimes even people in the shade get a tan. Even if it is cloudy, sunburn can still occur. Canopies, trees, and umbrellas do not offer complete protection. Drink plenty of water to avoid dehydration.

THE EYES

They say the eyes are the windows to the soul. Having perfectly healthy eyes, good vision, and being free of pain are essential to your health and well-being.

According to the Centers for Disease Control and Prevention (CDC), approximately 21 million Americans have numerous types of vision problems. Some are somewhat benign, like nearsightedness, but others, like glaucoma and age-related macular degeneration, can trigger vision loss and blindness.

The risk of developing an eye condition increases with age. African Americans and people with relative history of glaucoma may have a greater risk of developing the disease. People with diabetes can develop a condition called diabetic retinopathy, which can damage their retinas.

Some of the most common symptoms of eye diseases are:

Vision loss due to blurriness
Irritation from discharge irritation
Lightening strikes
Sensitivity to light
Seasonal allergies

The most common eye issues in the United States are classified as refractive errors, such as myopia (nearsightedness), hyperopia (farsightedness), astigmatism (blurry vision), and presbyopia (an inability to focus on objects up close). Most of these problems can be corrected with eyeglasses, contacts, or surgery.

Advanced serious eye conditions can eventually lead to loss of vision or blindness. Some of these diseases are age-related macular degeneration, cataracts, diabetic retinopathy, and glaucoma.

Here are some eye issues you can develop:

Refractive errors

Cataracts

Macular degeneration

Glaucoma Conjunctivitis

Optic neuritis is inflammation of the optic nerve.

Retinal diseases, such as a retinal tear or detachment,

Diabetic eye problems, such as diabetic retinopathy and diabetic macular edema,

The NIH National Eye Institute states that getting a dilated eye exam is simple and painless, and it's the single best thing you can do for your eye health!

Getting older raises the possibility of several eye diseases. You may possibly have a higher risk of eye illness if you:

Are you overweight?

A family history of eye disease

Are you African American, Native American, or Hispanic?

Safeguard your eyes

Wear sunglasses.

Wear sunglasses that block 99 to 100 percent of UVA and UVB radiation, even on cloudy days, to protect your eyes from the sun!

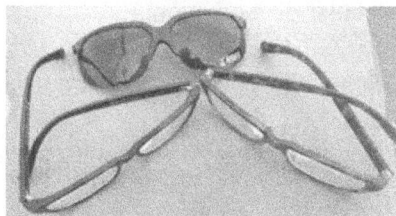

Wear protective eyewear.

Wear protective safety glasses or goggles to guard your eyes during activities like sports, production work, or home maintenance.

Rest your eyes -Working at a computer or a blackboard for a long time can tire out your eyes. Rest your eyes every 30 minutes and look at something about 30 feet away for 15 seconds.

If you wear contacts, you should take precautions to avoid eye infections.

Wash your hands before you place or take out your contact lenses, disinfect your contact lenses, and replace them regularly.

Tips for eye health:

Visit your eye doctor every one to two years.

Wear sunglasses when outdoors.

Wear protective eye gear when practicing sports, home projects, or work-related activities.

Control your blood sugar.

Training Concepts

Bodybuilding is a way to develop muscle mass, shape, and symmetry using progressive weights.

As you get stronger, you add more weight and your muscles grow in size and shape. Developing your own body requires knowledge about exercises, diets, nutrition, concentration, and balance.

Repetition or Reps

Bodybuilding usually focuses on sets and repetitions. Repetitions, or "reps," are the number of times you do an exercise. Always rest for a few minutes between sets, more if you are working out for mass with heavy poundage.

Sets

A set is when you do an exercise for various reps. For example, 1 set of 10 reps = 1 exercise repeated 10 times.

The Correct Weight

Select heavy weights for at least 6 to 8 reps and then continue forcing reps to 12. Don't use too heavy of a weight or too light. If you can do more than 10 or 12 reps, it is too light.

You should get to the last two reps with effort; keep adding resistance to continue growing. This is the concept of weight resistance. So remember to make progress, add weight. When the rep becomes easy to do, it is time to add weight, and the cycle repeats itself over and over again.

As you grow stronger and progress in strength and size, your training should become more and more intense. Then, as you continue to progress, you could adopt a split routine. That is when you work out some body parts one day and the other body parts the next day.

THE BASIC EXERCISES ARE:

- Deadlifting

- Curls

- The bench press

- Barbell press:

- Squats

1 or 2 abdominal exercises, like crunches or reverse crunches

Warm-up

Remember to always, warm-up; don't turn your warm-up into your workout. I personally use the Pyramid Principle. For example, I'll go x number of pounds for x number of reps and I'll go up in weight every set. Then I'll go down. That is my warm-up and exercise set.

Cool down

Cooling down is important because it releases lactic acid that gathers in the muscles during a hard training session, helping reduce the stuffiness and soreness after training. Never sit down after working out. Walk slowly and move your arms and neck to cool down.

Free Weights vs. Machines

My personal opinion, like many other champions, is that there is nothing like barbells and dumbbells. I believe free weights are better and more demanding on the muscles than machines or cables. One of the advantages of free weights is price. Don't get me wrong now; there are some machine exercises that are as good as or better than free weights. Of course, machines are safer; I also use machines in my workout. If you can, use both. Both have their good points.

Muscle Bound.

Not so long ago, people would say you were muscle-bound (lack of flexibility) if you developed your body using weights. Not true. Nowadays, football players, baseball players, boxers, and other athletes use weight resistance to get in shape. I think that old tale is over with.

Personal Log

I know people like Frank Zane, Mike Mentzer, and others used to write down everything that had to do with their training. They used it as feedback, so they didn't have to memorize everything.

Keeping a diary will help you keep track of your exercises, weights, reps, progress, and the foods you eat. It's also a good idea to take pictures to monitor progress. I have kept my log for about 10 years.

Support for the Back

Use a belt when doing doing heavy weight.

Wraps

Most people use wraps, especially if they have weak or injured joints. They use it on their knees and elbows when they're doing heavy exercises.

Bandana

Use one to prevent perspiration from getting into your eyes.

Hand Gloves

Many of today's bodybuilders use gloves. Gloves will help you with the grip.

This is all right, but I personally don't use them.

The Gym

Find one that is close to your home. Many people don't feel like driving especially too long, after a hard day's work. Make sure there is adequate equipment including machines and free weights, plenty of space and it's well ventilated.

Check the shower, make sure it's clean .It should also not be over crowded. Parking lot is something to keep in mind.

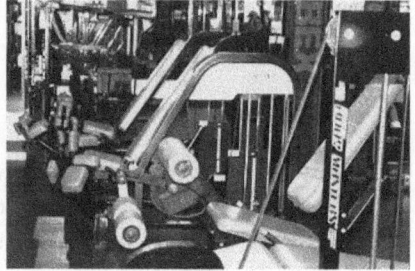

Home Gym

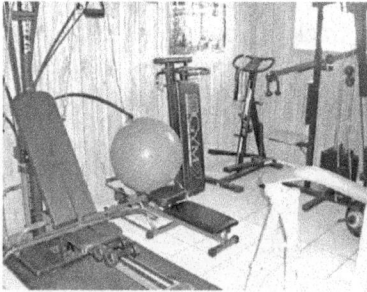

The Author home gym

You can develop a great body working out at home. Some champions, like Lou Ferrigno, used to train at home. Space should be one of the first requirements. You also need a bench that changes position, a barbell and two dumbbells at least, and if possible, an exercise machine. An exercise bike or a 'treadmill will be great. Make sure there is good ventilation.

Aerobics

Activity that relies on the intake of oxygen for energy.

Clothes

Loose-fitting clothes are a good idea. This is your choice, of course. Training in a cold room can be problematic if it's too cold.

Wear something warm to keep the body's heat, like a warm suit, sweatpants, and a sweatshirt.

Rubberized suits

I see a lot of people using it. They can endanger their lives. So please be careful. Sweating burns calories, yes, but it's a dangerous way to do it. Don't use it.

The best time to train

Choose a time that you can work out with no interruptions. This is your time. Let no obstacle stop you from training on the days you have chosen. Give your training time your undivided attention.

Overtraining

If you feel tired the next day, can't sleep well, or are not making the progress you expected, then maybe you are over training. Watch out!

The pump

When you train, you fill a muscle with blood, so your muscle appears larger. People described this feeling with all kinds of different remarks. This is the famous pump, and you can get addicted to it.

Burning

After an intense contraction exercise, you may experience a burning sensation and pain.

Muscle Pain:

This is common the day after a nice heavy workout. Many people are so sore the next day that they can't even get out of bed to go to work or even walk. If it hurts, stop! Find another exercise that works for you.

Dimensions

For size, use the basic exercises: bench press, squats, chins, rowing, seated press, and dead lift. Heavy weight with extra calories and proteins will make you gain size.

Explanation

To achieve definition, you have to combine nutrition, weights, cardiovascular stimulation, raising your heartbeat, and breathing.

Of course, using more calories for fuel will also help you lose fat. You can do it by restricting your carbohydrate intake, but many others swear by calories. Many people think that achieving maximum definition is a mystery. If you decide to remove carbohydrates, make sure to eat some so you have energy to train and do your cardio. You must reduce your body fat to at least 7% in order for veins and muscles to be visible.

Cardiovascular Exercise

Cardiovascular exercises are steady and non-stop. They should last at least 15 minutes and maintain the heart at 70 or 80% of your maximum heart rate. Proper breathing during exercise is important. Try to breath between repetitions, usually a gulp of air before the hardest part, but never hold it. There is no doubt that cardiovascular exercise is extremely important for a strong heart. When you do it, your heart beats faster and you breathe in more oxygen.

This extra stress makes the heart pump blood through your blood vessels. Like any other muscle, it must be used. How do you know when you've done enough? By monitoring your own pulse for 6 seconds and then adding a zero. For example, 13 beats plus zero equals 130 beats.

Personally, I know when I'm having a vigorous workout. The symptoms are clear; my heart is beating faster, my breathing is deeper, and I'm sweating more.

Cardio, when done correctly, will not only burn calories and fat while working, but will also burn calories and fat for hours after work. Muscle burns more energy than fat. Walking is a safe and simple cardiovascular exercise for all ages. Bicycling is also really good. Use of a treadmill inside the gym to walk or run is much safer, and it doesn't matter what the weather is like outside.

Try it. Some others are rowing, playing tennis, basketball, etc.

A recent report indicates that men with higher cardiorespiratory fitness levels are four times less likely to develop prostate cancer than men with low cardiorespiratory fitness levels. This same study also states that men who are physically active have a lower incidence of prostate cancer than men who are less active.

Nutrition

Nutrition plays a big role in bodybuilding. Eat healthy. Check the chapter on nutrition. You want to be big? Eat like a big man.

Yo-yo dieting

The definition of yo-yo dieting in the dictionary is the practice of going on slimming diets and putting the weight back on.

Relaxation

When you are stressed out, the first thing that happens to your body is something that you don't need. Adrenaline production shoots out, causing the fat cells from all over to move into your bloodstream so they can be used as energy. At the same time, your body is producing another hormone called "cortisol." Somehow it gets stored in the belly as fat.

Attitude

A positive attitude is of real importance for losing body fat or gaining muscle weight.

Stress Symptoms

Stress-related symptoms could include diarrhea, constipation, palpitations, anxiety, sleeplessness, skin problems, hair loss, and many other conditions.

Rest

Unless the body has ample time to recover through rest, the risk of injury increases. Rest is incredibly important to any fitness routine.

Humor

Humor is extremely good for your health. Most women love men with a good sense of humor. Men who smile a lot have better personalities, better health, less anxiety, less tension.

Laughing does wonders for digestion, lowers blood pressure, and keeps you optimistic and boosts your self-confidence.

Genetics

Genetics is heredity passed down from generation to generation, like blue eyes. Keep in mind that genetics will limit your own body development, no doubt about it!

Concentration

Concentrate when you are working out. Concentrate on your muscles. I believe that your mind can help your muscles grow through concentration. Do it!

Breathing deeply

Don't strain! Never, I repeat, never hold your breath when you are doing heavy training. At any time, Try to exhale when you are moving the weight into the hardest part.

Sleeping

Diabetes, heart disease, obesity, and high blood pressure have all been related to a lack of appropriate sleep. It is recommended to sleep at least 7–8 hours a day of uninterrupted sleep for maximum growth and reparation. This is up to you. Everybody is different.

Aging

You are as old as you feel. That is the truth. Well, there is no reason not to develop a nice body in your 40's, 50's, or even 60's. If you are older, you will develop muscles more slowly. If you are 40, 50, or older, I'm sure with the proper training you can develop a body that will be the envy of men half your age.

Working Out Partners

A training partner must use the same routine no matter the weight used. Having a partner is great because there are days when you don't feel like working out and your partner motivates you and pushes you.

Safety

Safety is very important in all the exercises you do, especially the squat and bench press. It is dangerous to work by yourself with heavy weights.

Precaution.

Always protect your elbows, shoulders, lower back, knees, and heels. If you injure any of these parts, your training will be held back or you will have to stop training for good. If at any time during your workout, it hurts, STOP! Find a different exercise to work out that muscle.

Gimmicks

There are always new gadgets on the market. Some have merit, but most of them are just a fast way to make a buck. There are no substitutes for barbells, dumbbells, or machines. Be alert.

It is not enough to know your craft-you have to have feeling.
Édouard Manet

Different specific Options

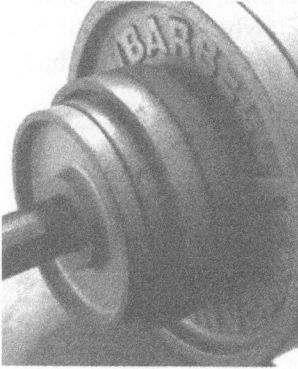

Weights Barbells are long bars with weights at each end. Dumbbells are smaller, hand-held weights.

Free weights are inexpensive and convenient.

Machines have the advantage of being safer and easier to use.

The disadvantage is that machines are not portable and can be expensive, so you may be limited to using exercise machines at a gym.

Stability balls These strength-training devices look like beach balls. The advantage of the stability ball is that it is inexpensive.

The disadvantage is that it is bulky and takes some space to keep.

Exercise bands or springs are portable and inexpensive. It is hard to progress. Many times, when you move from one band or spring to the next, it is very hard to do.

Kettlebells -Kettlebells were invented in Russia; they can be used for strength training and aerobic exercise, and they work all muscle groups at the same time.

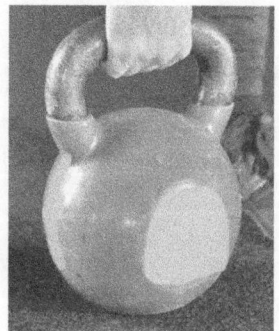

It looks like a cannonball with a handle. It is expensive. A workout with a kettlebell is high-intensity and involves a full range of motion.

Aerobic exercise- callisthenic own body weight.

Isometric

An isometric contraction is a static action where the muscle creates force, but there is no movement. Isometrics, like planks, pushing against a wall don't require you to move or bend any joints.

Generally, our contractions are stronger in our isometric contractions.

Eccentric

An eccentric contraction happens when the force generated by the muscle is less than the resistance, so the muscle actively lengthens. For example, when you are doing a biceps curl in the downward movement, its length increases. Generally, we are the second strongest in the eccentric phase.

Concentric

A concentric contraction happens when a muscle's force is superior to the resistance, so the muscle shortens; an example is in the upward phase of a bicep curl.

Finally, we are generally weakest in the concentric phase of a lift.

Isotonic exercise

Strengthen and build muscles so you can move through all types of motion with greater ease. These are the exercises that most people do in a gym. Like swimming, walking, and tennis.

Isokinetic exercise

This is a type of workout that involves machines that are not often used by the average person. It is mostly used by professional athletes to improve their sports.

Power

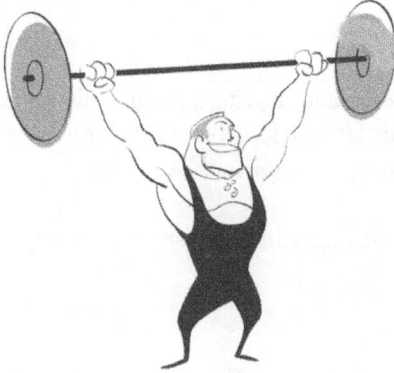

Power is speed and strength combined; I think explosive power training develops both. If you perform explosive training, you will probably become more agile and you will develop balance and coordination. Keep repetitions low, like 5 or 6, but you must do them very fast and in an explosive way.

Of course, remember that you must **always** warm up first. If you notice pain in the knees, your low back, or elbows, stop and try another exercise or routine.

Plyometrics (plyos)

Training using speed and force with different movements It includes exercises like running, jumping, push-ups, and kicking.

Many athletes use this training method to get in shape for sports like basketball, soccer, and baseball, as well as fighters.

The disadvantage is the risk of injuries, with the stress and strain placed on your knees when you jump and land.

Callisthenics

Exercises are performed rhythmically and generally with no equipment. They are body-weight training, aimed at promoting fitness, developing muscle tone, and are often used to lose weight and get in shape.

Cross-training

Cross-training is used for fitness purposes like endurance, strength, flexibility, and muscle development.

Many professional athletes perform cross-training as part of their routines. Activities are aerobic, strength training, endurance, and balance.

Circuit training

Circuit training is a fast-paced exercise; you perform one exercise for 30 seconds to 3 minutes, then move on to another exercise. When one circuit is finished, you begin the first exercise again for the next circuit. It consists of both aerobic exercise and strength training.

You do eight to 10 different exercises, like a stationary bike, weight machine, or a jump rope.

Interval training

During interval training, you tax your heart and then let it recover while you keep working at a less intense level. You train until you are almost breathless, then you return to your level but without resting. This is called active recovery.

Sprints

Sprints and other high-intensity bursts of cardio are excellent for conditioning and aid in fat loss while maintaining muscle mass.

Group exercise classes

High impact: High impact is defined as an exercise when both feet leave the ground at the same time.

Low impact cardiovascular is when one foot remains on the ground.

They are combinations of the two mentioned above.

Weight training and bodybuilding

Bodybuilders use weight training to develop muscle size, shape, and symmetry for bodybuilding contests; the idea is to maximize muscular size and obtain extremely low levels of body fat.

The basis of the bodybuilding system is the number of repetitions (reps), sets, tempo, exercise types, and weight to cause an increase in size and definition.

Strength training is essential in sports that require it.

Bodybuilding, weightlifting, powerlifting, football, and many other sports use strength training as part of their training routine.

Workouts advance systems

Reps cheated

When you can no longer execute a given number of reps, you add just enough body momentum and assistance from other muscles to keep the weight moving.

Single-set resting after each exercise.

The Supersets

You select two exercises and perform them back to back, with no rest between them; you do one for a specific muscle group and the other for an opposing muscle group.

Tri-sets

Three exercises are done one after the other with no rest.

Rest and pause.

When you complete your desired reps, you rest for a few seconds, do a rep or two, rest, and do one more rep.

Pre-exhaustion

You perform an isolation exercise first to fatigue the primary muscle, and then you do a compound movement.

Pyramid System

You decrease the reps as you increase the weight, then after you get to use heavy weight, you begin lowering the weight and increase the reps. Mr. Olympia-Mr. Universe Sergio Oliva told me he used this system many times in his career.

Negatives

You reach your final reps, and your training partner helps you raise the weight to the top position, then you lower the weight in a controlled manner.

Partials

You don't do a full rep or movement, you stop or do a partial rep.

"Never put off till to-morrow what you can do to-day"
Tomas Jefferson

Gyms rules

Most gyms have rules and regulations, and most of them have signs posted with the rules. Most are common sense.

Examples of rules to be followed are:

1. Time restrictions on a machine

2-Be patient when waiting to use a particular machine.

3-Clean out your sweat from a machine with a towel after using one.

4-When there is a line waiting to take a sip at the water fountain, don't fill your water bottle.

Remember, there is a code of conduct in every gym.

Gym essentials in a bag

1-Towel–to wipe out your own sweat and wipe out the sweat from a machine.

2-Some gyms give you a key when you arrive, and you return it when you leave. Some gyms ask you for your driver's license or other kind of ID and return it to you when you turn the key in before you leave.

3-Shoes: shower shoes if you are planning to take a shower or get into the sauna.

4-Water bottle

5) Shorts are ideal for allowing a full range of motion.

6-T-shirt-A comfortable one-If you're a woman, a sports bra.

If it is cold, you should wear a sweat shirt during exercise, but more importantly, after you work out and you are sweaty.

Choosing a gym

First considerations: price, location (distance from home or work), Member capacity: is it crowded? You don't want to wait all the time to move from one piece of equipment to the next.

Hours: Knowing the time you are going to be able to go is important. Parking-enough space? Equipment: enough equipment? Quality, condition, well maintained?

Regulars: Are the people attending nuisances? Loud? Cleanliness: Is it clean? What about the showers? The gym floor? Management attitude: Do you feel they are only after you?

Why pay more? If you are not going to use special facilities. Do people come to this gym to workout or socialize?

Exercise Classes

Aerobics can be hard on some people's joints; low-impact classes are better.

Kickboxing is an outstanding way to get in shape. You will learn some self-defense moves while you are getting in shape.

Steps (Aerobics): You use a small bench or block to step up and down.

Plyometric: These exercises are done in a very explosive way, with short bursts of power jumps. Excellent body conditioning.

Personal trainers

These trainers guide you through the exercises and equipment, and they help you move the weight to the barbell bar or machine. They keep you enthusiastic. My son was one for many years. If you are planning to hire one, choose one that has a legitimate credential from a fitness organization.

Gym Equipment

You could buy and use most of these machines at home.

Elliptical Cross trainer

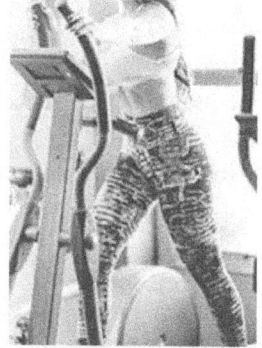

These machines are intended to make joint work easier. You burn calories on one of these machines just as if you were jogging, but with less stress on your joints. In my opinion, and the opinion of many others, they are very tiresome preventing you from getting a good workout

Treadmill

The Treadmill is one, if not the most popular exercise device for cardiovascular training.
Designed to give you a great cardio workout by walking or running, it is excellent for use when it is raining or cold outside. Some adjust the height and the speed, from slow walking to sprinting.

Stationary Bicycles

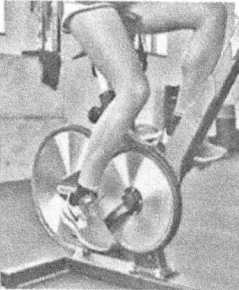

Exercise bikes: Exercise bikes: There are different kinds of bicycles. More than any other piece of equipment, stationary upright bikes are used for physical rehabilitation. They are low-impact on your joints and, at the same time, offer excellent cardiovascular exercise.

You can exercise at a long-slow-distance pace or go for high intensity intervals.

They take up less space than a treadmill, which can be an important consideration in a small apartment or home. Recumbent bikes are the ones you pedal with your feet in front instead of down. Experts claim these are easy on your knees and joints. Personally, I don't like them. Upright bikes allow you to ride like a regular bike.

Steppers

Some people call them stair climbers. The pedal adjusts to various resistance levels. It is a great lower body exercise. You work your buttocks, legs, and calves. I personally don't like this machine.

Rowing machine

This machine was designed to give you an upper body and a cardiovascular workout. It mimics the motion of a rowing boat. Rowers are excellent for cardiovascular exercise, and they are also good for building muscles as well.

They are low-impact and work both your upper and lower body during each complete rowing stroke. This machine is fantastic.

Machine for lifting weights

The Machines benefits are that these machines are much safer than free weights. If you stop, for whatever reason, the weight is not going to come crashing down on you.

The weight selection is easy to change compared to a regular barbell. Just move a pin to select a weight change. Also, it is compact, so you save a lot of space.

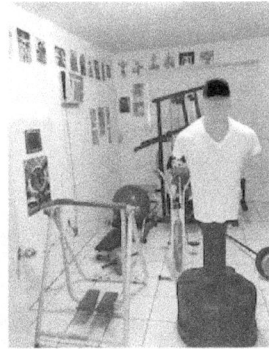
Author home gym

These are the most popular machines you are going to find in a gym or in a home gym. You can get a good workout by training with free weights, free exercises, machines, and other kinds of apparatus. You must concentrate on the major muscles like the legs and back. The core muscles around your center are important to train because they stabilize the body.

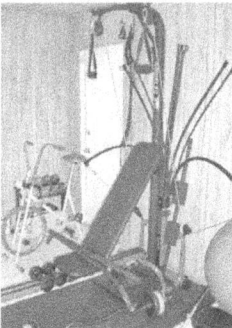
Author home gym

51

Sergio Oliva

During the 60's, I was a skinny young guy, walking home from school when suddenly, it happened. I saw Sergio Oliva on a magazine cover at a newsstand and bought the magazine. The man in the picture was humongous, with perfect proportions, long muscles, and incredible symmetry. From that moment on, I wanted to train and to look like him.

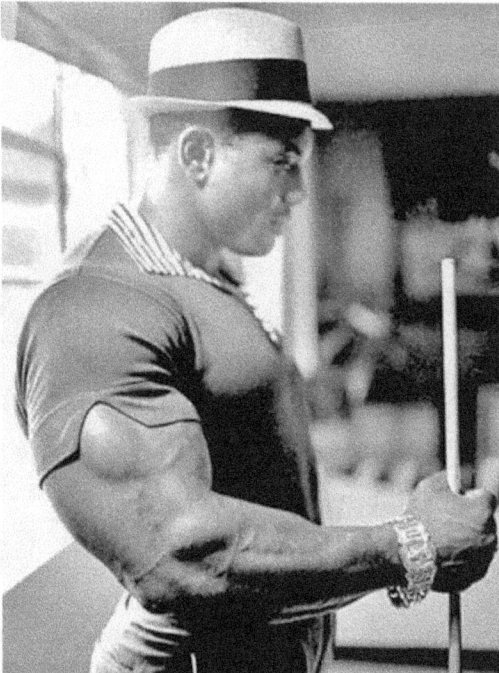

The way he inspired me, he inspired thousands of others. That is how I met Sergio Oliva.

Sergio possessed the most superior, favorable genetics of all bodybuilders. He won many major competitions.

They called him THE MYTH, and he certainly lived up to those attributes.

When Sergio visited Arthur Jones in Florida, Arthur measured his arms vs. his head and found out his arms were bigger than his head. Arthur claimed that no one else in history could make that claim.

Sergio lived his life like the song "My Way" or "His Way" without compromising one single value. He always stood tall for the truth he believed in, no matter the price he had to pay.

"From the Introduction of the book by Sergio Oliva the Myth book"

He became legendary not only for winning so many titles and having one of, if not the, greatest physiques of all time, with his perfect, massive, symmetrical body, without ever wavering from his beliefs, but also for standing up to the establishment, refusing to endorse fraudulent supplements he did not believe in, and refusing to sell to the public anything other than his own integrity.

Sergio is the inspiration for the manga character Biscuit Oliva from the Martial Arts Manga series Baki. In the series, he is one of the strongest men in the world, unstoppable (his nickname is "The Unchained"), and he chases dangerous criminals around the world, making a close bond of friendship and rivalry with Baki and Yuujiro, "the strongest creatures in the world."

I met Sergio many times personally and spoke to him for countless hours over the phone. He was my teenage idol. He was a very knowledgeable and charismatic man, and I enjoyed all the conversations and anecdotes he told me.

I'm proud and honored that Sergio picked me to write his only book, Sergio Oliva the Myth. I will always have a place in my heart for Sergio.

From The Sergio Oliva the Myth book dedication

"If you work then you deserve it."
Sergio Oliva

Arthur Jones-Vince Gironda-Mike Mentzer

Influence in training -Vince Gironda

Besides Sergio Oliva, the Myth, Vince Gironda, Arthur Jones, and Mike Mentzer have been the biggest influences on me. I read everything I could find about them, including books and articles, and I practiced and learned everything I could from them.
I believe, along with many other experts in the field, that no trainer in the history of bodybuilding has brought more controversial thinking and training concepts than Vince, Arthur, and Mike.

If an actor needed to get into shape, where did he/she go? Of course, they went to Vince Gironda, he was referred to as "The Trainer of the Stars", and among his clients were Clint Eastwood, Cher, Michael Douglas, Robert Blake, and others, he was an individual ahead of his time, and many call him the Iron Guru.

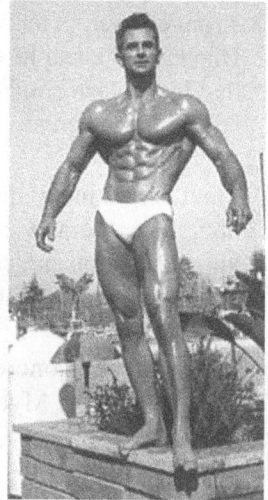

Gironda was not a public relations kind of guy. *Vince Gironda*
One of the many stories surrounding Vince goes like this: When Arnold came to America and went to see Vince, he presented himself in an arrogant way. Gironda told him, "Well, you look like a fat fuck to me." Gironda's gym members and associates described him as unpredictable, rude, and impossible to work with. He was famous for kicking people out of his gym for going against exercises he was against like, bench press, squats etc.

In 1972 Vince created his own nutritional supplements called NSP. Gironda was against the use of steroids for physique development, he said it will give you a grotesque appearance.
Some of his ideas were so revolutionary that some people did not want to accept them. He trained Larry Scott one of his most famous pupil, Larry won the first 2 Mr. Olympia contest.

He created a specials shoulder press for Larry Scott to develop his shoulders and he called it Scott press. For biceps he recommended the Preacher curl-he name it the "Scott Curls".

He had many theories, like why he was against bodybuilders doing squats because they would develop the glue and hips. He recommended doing sissy squats instead. For training the calves he insisted that calves raises should be done barefoot and high reps, with a full range of motion. For the back Vince recommended using full motion range like touching the sternum to the bar when doing chinning to complete contract the latissimus muscles.

He also believed that aerobics would compromise muscle mass, which, according to him, meant slow fat loss, and that weight training was superior for women to lose body fat. The abdominal-he concludes that there were more misunderstandings concerning this muscle than any other body part. He believed, through his experience, that daily abdominal work produced a smooth look, loss of muscle tone, and a bloating effect. Due to immense hormone loss.

Gironda also popularized the diet Maximum Definition Diet 40 years ago or more, eating only fats and protein for three to four days straight, followed by one day of only carbohydrates. Most people know it today as the Atkins diet. It was an incredible approach because it became the diet of many champions, like Arnold, Dave Draper, Larry Scott, and many more. "It was just called meat and eggs."

Creating an illusion: cosmetic bodybuilding.

Vince believed in creating illusions. To him, everything was about shape, symmetry, and balancing proportions with classical lines, reducing and building up certain areas to transform the way you look in a fantastic way. Vince called it "cosmetic bodybuilding." Many people's only concern is putting on weight, no matter where they are or how much they can lift, no matter where it goes or the way they end up looking. Vince was only concerned with having a symmetrical body and achieving Greek proportions.

In 1980, MuscleMag International -Robert Kennedy publisher in collaboration with Vince published a book title "Unleashing the Wild Physique". It contained Vince knowledge through his 30+ experience.

Some myths and facts, according to Vince:

It's a myth that abdominal exercises are fat emulsifiers and reducers.

It's a myth that abdominal exercises produce a small waist.

It's a myth that eating fat causes you to get fat. On the contrary, fat burns fat.

It's a myth that side bends reduce the waistline.

It's a fact that side bends build muscles and thicken the waist.

It's a fact that squats build the glutes and the waist,

It's a fact that swimming makes you fat.

It's a myth that bench presses build pecs. It's a deltoid exercise.

It's a fact that bodybuilding is 85% nutrition.

He opposed:

Mixing carbohydrates with protein.
Skipping breakfast.
Lack of concentration during workouts

Former magazine editor/writer and photographer Denie Walter gave him. "The Iron Guru" a name.

I've adopted many of Vince's techniques and theories; he was and still is one of the biggest influences on my own philosophy today.

"Remember that nutrition is 90%; exercise is 10%".
Vince Gironda

Arthur Jones

Arthur Allen Jones, a wild animal enthusiast, inventor, exercise philosopher, and film maker, produced a TV series called "Wild Cargo" was the founder of Nautilus, Inc. and MedX, Inc. medical-based exercise equipment for the cervical spine, lumbar spine, and knee. Jones was interested in improving the lives of geriatric patients in nursing homes and was the inventor of the Nautilus exercise machines during the 70's and 80's.

Jones began training with a barbell when he was 12 years old; he was an incredibly smart and amazing man. This put him on the Forbes list of the 400 richest people. Financial analysts estimated he was grossing $400 million annually. Jones was born in 1924 in Arkansas and grew up in Tulsa, Okla. The son of two physicians, he dropped out of school in the ninth grade, declaring that he had assimilated all he needed from the education system.

Arthur developed Jumbolair Aviation Estates in Ocala, whose most notable resident is actor John Travolta. Arthur taught himself how to fly, was an accomplished pilot, and owned and flew several jetliners. Jones had on his property 90 elephants, 300 alligators, 400 crocodiles, a gorilla, three rhinos, and many poisonous snakes and insects. Jones was married six times; most of his wives were aged 16 to 20 years old.

Jones transformed the fitness industry, transforming the gyms into the fashionable fitness clubs popular today. Joe Moore, president of the International Health, Racquet & Sports Club Assn., said, "Many of the innovations he came up with in the 1970s are still incorporated into strength training on machines of all brands."

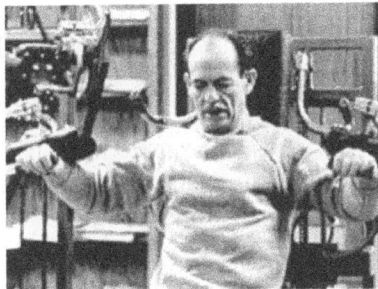

Arthur Jones

He popularized the pre-exhaustion system, Arthur Jones believed that it was the best way to train; it is a brutally hard system. He had about 50 patents under his name.

He wrote articles for all of the health and bodybuilding magazines of the time, including articles for Sport Illustrated 1975, New Body 1982, People 1983, Playboy 1983, Science Digest 1984, Time 1985, Macleans 1985, and Club Industry 1994. Sport Illustrated wrote in 1975 that those Jones machines were being used by wrestlers, college football teams, NFL teams, and star athletes.

Arthur Jones forever changed exercise and rehabilitative medicine with his concept of "train hard, train briefly, train infrequently." He believed that you either train hard or you can train for a long time, but you can't do both. A workout can be hard or a workout can be long. There is no such thing as a long and hard workout.

One of the many stories surrounding Arthur goes like this: When Arthur first met Arnold, Jones he pulled the car over, walked out to the other side, and threatened to kick Arnold's ass right there if he didn't stop running his mouth. He thought that "Arnold was someone that couldn't train hard if his life depended on it.

He sold Nautilus Inc. in 1986 for $23 million. He also sold MedX Corporation in 1996 and then retired. He died on August 28, 2017 of natural causes in his home in Ocala, Florida at age 80.

Jones, a tough man who used to carry a gun, claimed that he "shot 630 elephants and 63 men, and he regretted the elephants more." His motto was "younger women, faster airplanes, and bigger crocodiles."

I'm glad and honored that I had the opportunity to talk over the phone with Arthur many times, and I'm grateful that he gave me permission to use some of his photographs.

"How old am I? Old enough to know it's impossible to change the thinking of fools, but young and foolish enough to keep on trying."

Arthur Jones

Mike Mentzer

Mike Mentzer was a legend in bodybuilding, the first person to ever earn a perfect 300 score in the Mr. Universe in Acapulco, Mexico. After he retired, Mike became a leading trainer, and had a regular monthly column "Heavy Duty" in Ironman magazine.

Mentzer took the concepts of Arthur Jones and worked to perfect them, thinking back over years of study and observations. He improved the principles of high-intensity training. Creating Heavy Duty, he insisted, like Jones, that training had to be brief, infrequent, and intense to get results

He concluded that if you decide to train the whole body in one day, starting with the largest muscles first, in descending or to the smallest, like the legs, back, chest, deltoids, and arms. The largest muscle group should always be trained first. This is why many champions, like Steve Reeves, work the whole body

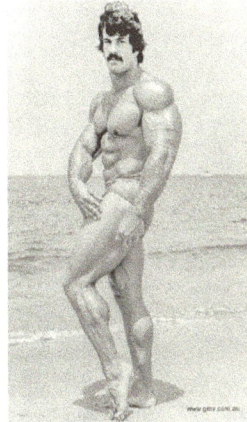

Zero rest time between exercises-cut workout time-train the entire body-never train more than four days a week.

Wayne Gallash photo

Select only 10 basic exercises or less; limit each exercise to two sets.

Perform each exercise in a high-intensity manner until no more reps are possible. Increase the weight whenever possible, but don't sacrifice technique. When you can do more than 6 reps, increase the weight.

Rey Mentzer (Mike brother) won 1979 AAU Mr. America; both were examples of excellent genetics.

"It is virtually impossible for the average man or woman to understand the extraordinary effort involved in building an Olympian physique".
Mike Mentzer

What Men and Woman Worry About

Adult Men	Body Part	Adult Women
17%	Natural hair	32%
21%	Gray hair	29%
24%	Thinning hair	18%
20%	Facial hair	27%
10%	Eyebrows	22%
9%	Nose	10%
4%	Lips	8%
11%	Wrinkles	28%
23%	Skin	40%
10%	Chin/neck	27%
8%	Arms	23%
7%	Hands	13%
9%	Nails	18%
15%	Excess body hair	15%
14%	Chest / Breasts	24%
52%	Stomach	69%
5%	Cellulite	29%
7%	Butt	29%
4%	Hips	25%
5%	Thighs	36%
5%	Legs	20%
2%	Ankles	5%
8%	Feet	12%
% likely to worry about/obsess over body part		

Warm-up

Your warm-up should not be very long, but it should be long enough. The length of a warm-up varies from person to person as well as with age. You will be preparing your body to go from a resting state to more activity. Of course, five minutes will be sufficient, of course, depending on your age, physical condition, and weather.

Warm-up reduces the risk of injuries and prevents you from getting strains, muscle pulls, etc. Your muscles, tendons, and ligaments need a gradual increase to accommodate the activity you will do.

My warm-ups consist of moving around, punching in the air, and a light set. Then I would go up in weight for the same exercise, making my warm-up part of my first sets.

For some people, the warm-up is more important than others. You have to learn this by yourself.

Find out how much warm-up you need and what works for you. Don't make it too long, just enough to save your energy for your heavy workout. Warm-ups are good, but keep them short and to the point.

Go Slowly

Losing weight slowly is the safest and correct way to redefine your body.

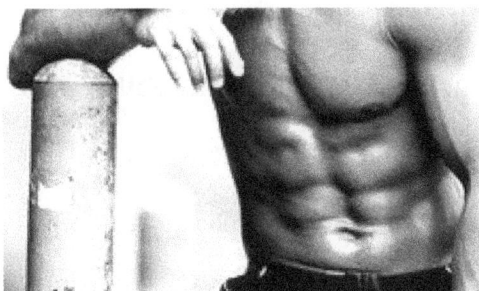

The idea of Arthur Jones, the inventor of Nautilus equipment, a writer and a genius bodybuilding expert, is to work as hard as you can for a short period of time.

Ease: Ease into your gym routine to avoid injuries.

Slow Down: Rushing during your workout puts you at risk of injury. Don't forget to breathe. Don't hold it.

Safety means a gradual increase in intensity to your regular workout. Warming up should give you an increase in range of motion that is specific to the activity you are about to perform. This is a must to reduce the risk of injury.

Rest: Taking a break between workouts is important. This is when your body recuperates from your workout. It is when your muscles grow and you gain strength. Not when you are working out.

Results Overnight: It takes time to add lean muscular weight to the body, and it may take weeks before you start to see results. Sometimes you don't see any for weeks, and then you wake up one day and all of a sudden. Wow!!!You will start to see a big change!

Cooling off

After a workout, you may experience some onset soreness or pain in your muscles. This is normal between 20 and 40 hours after exercising. If you keep exercising, this will disappear in a few days.

Always stretch at the end of a workout:

Take a couple of minutes to stretch; I always do it at the end of a workout.

Recovery Situations: Rest:

Do not work out if you feel tired.

I have not had a good night's sleep in at least 48 hours.

Females: in the first days of your monthly cycle, especially during heavy cycles.

When you have cold-like symptoms, such as the flu, your body needs to rest.

Early AM Exercises

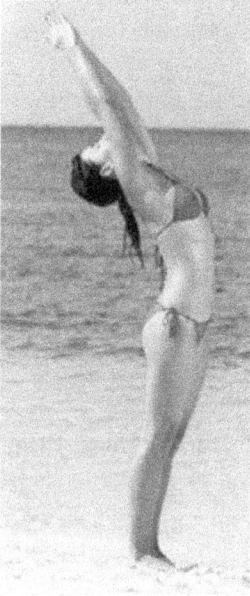

If it is convenient, try to run, walk, and exercise in the morning. The ancient Romans and Greeks used the Latin term "Carpe Diem," meaning "do the necessary work before noontime." This is important for the following reasons:

The air is purer.

During the summer months, it is cooler in the morning, providing more privacy and quiet.

Boost your metabolism for the day.

Your workout is finished. You can go about your day, and you will feel energetic for the rest of the day.

Here are some ideas to dress correctly:

Wear loose clothes.
A good pair of running shoes
Dress coolly in the summer.
Dress warmly during the winter months. Sweat pants, sweat shirts, wind breaker, gloves and hat are all important articles of clothing.

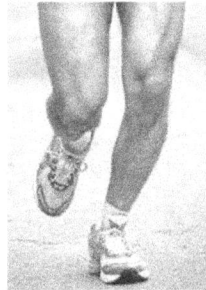

AM

It is my belief, and those of many others, that exercise in the morning makes your metabolism speed up and stay up for part of the whole day.

Follow tips below:

Stretch, go for a 5-minute walk with your dog; anything you do in the morning will improve your circulation and energy level.

Select Wisely: Try to eat a moderate breakfast. Eat something healthy. Don't be a slave. Have a glass of milk, fruit, and a wheat piece of bread.

Check the local weather report before any outdoor activity so you can choose the appropriate number of layers, or rain coat. If you use any headphones with your CD player or MPs, keep the volume low to be able to hear surrounding noises like car horns, dog barking, or people approaching.

Try to exercise throughout the day; try real-life workouts: Bring your groceries to the car; don't use the elevator. Park a few blocks from your destination and use the stairs.

Your action expresses your priorities.
Mahatma Gandhi

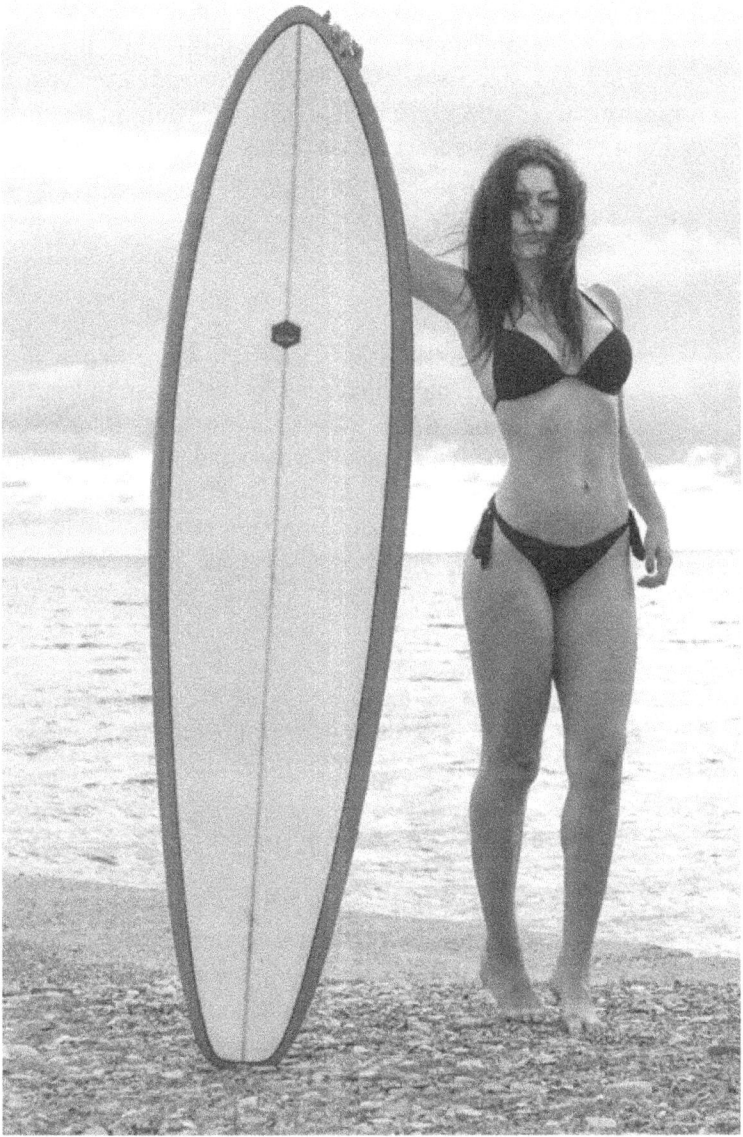

Photo by Igor Starkov

Exercising

Exercise not only gives you a lean and strong body, but also decreases heart disease, diabetes, and colon cancer. Exercise maintains strong bones, muscles, and joints and relieves arthritis pain. It's excellent for your mind, too, since it relieves stress. Your body uses your body fat for energy to complete an exercise session. It doesn't matter if you are taking a brisk walk or working out at the gym. The good thing about exercise is that it builds muscles and burns calories even when you're at rest. This is terrific!!

Sleep

A recent American Heart Association study found that those who practice healthy sleep habits have a 42% lower risk of heart failure than those who do not. Sleep will make you feel and look younger, and it will also make you mentally sharp and physically strong. For me, 5 or 5 hours of sleep is all I need. You have to discover it for yourself. But don't ignore this. Your body can't go too long without sleeping. During sleep, the heart rate lowers, the digestive and circulatory systems rest and repair. They don't stop working, they just slow down.

I know some people take muscle naps for 5 or 10 minutes every day. It works great for them. This is something I have never done myself. However, you might experiment and see what happens.

The atmosphere

Fresh air is essential to your health. The air invigorates and regenerates your whole body. Breathe fresh air anytime you can, at the beach or at the park. Think about it: we spend most of our time inside four walls at work, at home, at school, at the mall, or at the theater, with air conditioning or a heater.

When I was a child, kids played baseball or other games outside, but now most kids in the city spend most of their time inside with video games, computers, etc.

The Truth about Fasted Cardio

Try to run in the morning if possible. Fasted morning cardio increases the amount of free fatty acids used up as fuel.

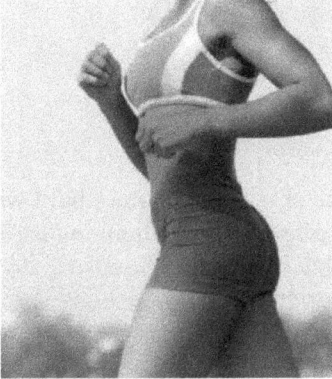

While sleeping, approximately 100% of the energy used comes from fatty acids because of the extremely low intensity of the activity; the natural HGH burst occurs approximately 30 minutes so when you enter the deep sleep phase (HGH increases fatty acid operation).

Later, fat is the main energy source during your sleeping period. Probabilities are that upon waking, you have a greater number of free fatty acids available.

Therefore, morning cardio in a fasted state could increase fat loss and allow a bodybuilder in a bulking phase to increase their carb intake without gaining more fat.

Cardio explanation

Numerous authorities believe that you lower your growth hormone when cardio is performed before weights, reducing muscle growth and strength.

Do cardio after weight training or if you can on another day.

A warm-up of three or four minutes at a slow pace, while walking or on a tread-mill, is all that is required.

Stay away from cardio in a bulk mass phase; do it only for a very short time as a warm-up.

The Truth about Fasted Cardio-Continuation

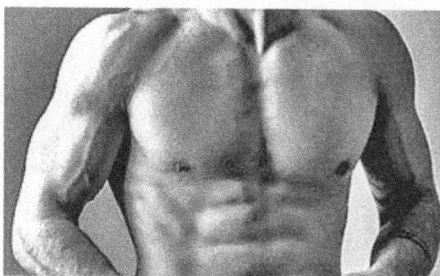

I personally believe in the importance of morning cardio, but I won't tell you that morning cardio is more effective than afternoon cardio. It works when it comes to fat loss. I think it is common sense to do light aerobic work before a weight workout, to warm up the body and prepare the mind for the work ahead.

I also believe that aerobic exercise after a grueling muscle-building workout would postpone the response to the body's need for nutrition, rest, and recuperation. So it's best to do aerobics on a day when you're not working. I'm a hard gainer. I love weight training and have been doing it since 1962, and I had to discover the best way to train the hard way.

This is the conclusion:
Don't use lengthy workouts.
Brief, hard, heavy training
Follow a balanced diet
Get adequate sleep and rest.
The goal is to increase poundage, short rest, less frequent training, more reps, low reps, vary the exercises, vary routines.

Diet

If you are attempting to lose weight, you should indulge yourself every 2 or 3 days with a treat. For example, if you go out with friends, share a couple of pizza slides, a sandwich, or a dinner, and you will feel great and have a good time. This trick works like a knockout.

Fasting

Most people don't know that when you fast, you also lose muscle along with fat. The truth is, anytime you fast, you lose muscle along with the fat. My grandfather used to have a partial fast every two weeks and a full fast once a month. He lived past 90 years with his mind and body in perfect working order, eating whatever he wanted and dancing until a week or two before he died. He swears by fasting.

He believed that fasting cleaned him of toxins. Sometimes he used to drink juices, but 95% of the time he used to fast with water alone. He claimed he could concentrate better and he felt great after each time he fasted.

Keep in mind that some people get sick or dizzy when fasting. When you finish with your fast, go back to eating and gradually take a day or two to eat your regular diet.

You should discuss it with your doctor if you are going to try it. In my case, I do a light fast once a year.

Dress

You must keep your muscles warm, especially if it is cool outside. A T-shirt and shorts are OK if it is summer or warm outside. If it is cold, wear a sweet shirt, a cap, or a hat. It is very important to keep warm on winter days.

"The future stars today, not tomorrow".
Pope John Paul II

Cardio to lose weight

If glycogen is available in your body for fuel, your body won't get it from body fat stores. This is why you should never eat or drink carbohydrates before cardio. Many experts believe, including myself, that the first cardio should be done when you wake up on an empty stomach or when there is no glycogen stored in your muscles if your goal is to lose fat and get hard. Fat burning is greatest during the first 15 minutes of exercise.

There are believers that say that morning cardio won't be significantly more effective than post-workout or afternoon cardio work when it comes to fat loss

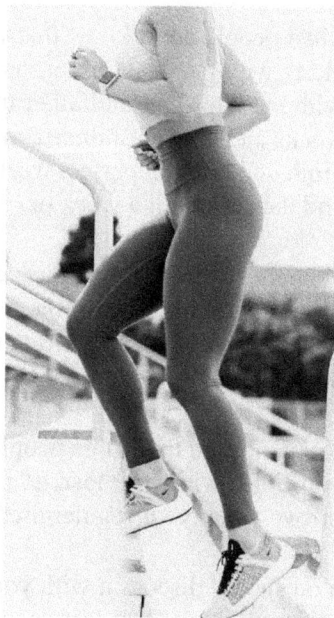

Step-ups

Cardio to put on weight

If your intention is to put on muscle and you're eating to maintain growth, it's counterproductive to break a sweat on the treadmill or go for a bike ride, right? Actually, no. Cardio holds many major benefits for individuals who wish to build a lean physique, and there are situations in which you should avoid it completely.

Your personal situation will dictate how much you need. For example, if you have some fat to shed, you'll want adequate sessions to facilitate that—up to three 45-minute steady-state workouts (like running, biking, at a consistent pace) or 15–30 minute high-intensity interval training (HIIT) sessions.

On the other hand, if you're a hard-gainer (a.k.a., skinny), you want just sufficient cardio to strengthen your heart and get the blood pumping to those hard-worked muscles to accelerate recovery. That could mean moderate-intensity 10-minute steady-state bouts as a bridge to your lifting routines.

<u>Tips to consider:</u>

Always wear loose clothes.

Always wear a good pair of shoes.

In the summer, dress to keep cool and comfortable.

In the winter, dress warmly. Sweat pants, sweat shirts, windbreakers, gloves, and hats are all important articles of clothing.

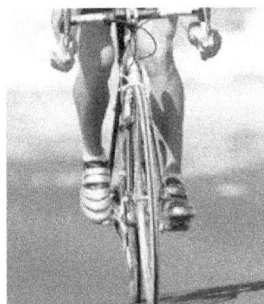

The goal is to increase pounds, short rest, less frequent workouts, more reps, low reps, change the exercises, change routines.

Rules

Train wise

Rest

Warning pain

For legs

Don't try to jerk the weight while doing a deadlift.
1 medium-sized set
1 large set

Cardio

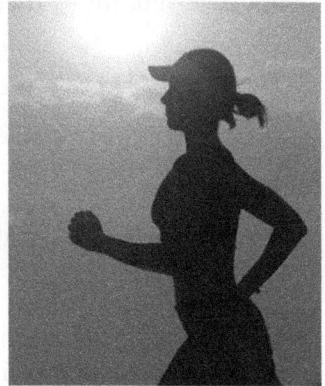

I do fast walking in the morning. If possible, I try to run or walk in the morning. Fast cardio increases the amount of free fatty acids (FFA) used as fuel. I believe morning cardio in a fasted state can boost fat loss.

I personally do believe in the efficacy of morning cardio, but not in a completely fasted state. I drank a small coffee cup before going out for my fast walk.

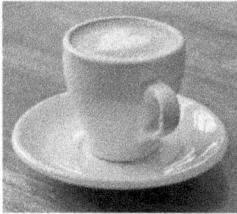

If your goal is to gain muscle bulk, you have to eat to stimulate growth. It's not smart to spend hours on the treadmill. Cardio helps people obtain a lean physique.

Doing cardio aerobics is good for people trying to lose fat.

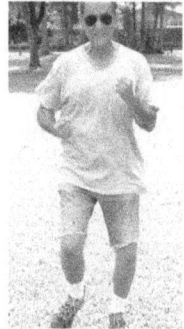

If you are skinny, you may think twice about doing cardio. You may do some for heart and lung conditioning, but never too much or too long.

I believe that too much running will interfere with your muscle building progress.

The Author early running

Aerobics are essential and valuable in your quest for physical fitness. If you run over an extended period on concrete, your knees might begin to show the strain, as well as your feet, ankles, and hips from all the pounding.

More data on cardio

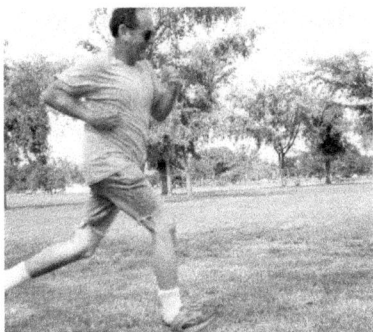

The author morning run

Every fitness magazine you open today has all kinds of experts giving their opinion on it. Should I do cardio? Cardiovascular exercise burns calories. Because burning calories promotes fat loss, experts think cardio is the answer. It makes sense, but it's more than that.

It takes a lot more work and determination to sculpt a lean body than cardio does. Most women and men trying to lose weight probably make one or more of these mistakes, if not more.

- Skips breakfast

- Overeats in the second half of the day

- It consumes too little protein.

- It makes meals way too far apart.

- Having the main meal at night

Running Backward

When I visit the park early in the morning, I always try to run backwards, at least for six minutes. Backward runners do not generate the same amount of pent-up energy as forward runners; instead, they use more leg muscles than forward runners and burn approximately 30% more energy to maintain the same pace.

Current studies show that running backwards improves fitness. Since it is relatively strenuous, backward running can be effective in building fitness. A study established that walkers' going backward results in excellent progress in physical performance compared to the amount of forward walking.

According to a recent study, professional runners who switched their usual training system for five weeks to backward running became approximately 2.5 percent more efficient when running forward by the end. They find out they can run faster without requiring more oxygen.

Research shows that backward running also causes less pounding of the knees, as research shows. On the downside, people often trip or slam into objects.

An authority study concluded that backward running results in "a higher magnitude of coordination variability" than forward running. The benefits can outweigh the risks, says Giovanni Cavagna, an emeritus professor of physiology at the University of Milan in Italy, who led the study. "Backward running allows training without repetitive pounding," he says.

It's best to try it first on a running track, he suggests, or with a forward-running partner who can point out obstacles.

Agility and Balance

<u>Balance-barefoot-eyes closed</u>

An amazing basic skill exercise for balance and ankle strength that I practice almost every day when I finish my cardio is standing and walking down the edge of a beam with control and balance.

Initially, you will walk slowly, but as you progress, you will be able to walk faster and then walk with your eyes closed on the wood edge beam or side walk edge.

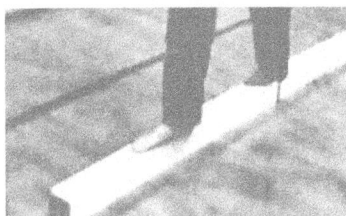

Make sure your beam or sidewalk edge is low enough in case you fall from it.

<u>Single leg stance: stand</u> on one leg with your arms crossed over your chest, maintaining a slight bend in the supporting leg for 10 seconds, if necessary, holding onto a chair or wall. As you progress, you can do it with your eyes closed. This helps the brain and body work together.

<u>Tightrope walking</u>: imagine a line in your path in front of you, then walk forward and place each foot on the imaginary line. As you adapt, try it with your eyes closed for a few seconds.

<u>Reverse walking</u> allows you to train all the senses in your body. This is reserved for outdoor walking. Walk backward, turn around, and walk forward for a few minutes. Repeat. As you adapt, walk with your eyes closed for a few seconds at a time.

<u>Walk forward</u>, pausing to balance on one of your legs, your supporting knees slightly bent. Lift one leg and touch your thigh on the supporting leg for a second, pointing the raised, bent knees to the side rather than forward. Keep your arms out for balance. To make it harder, raise your palms overhead and touch them. This yoga exercise will stretch your back muscles and give you stability and balance.

Aerobic Exercises

Walking

The easiest and simplest of the aerobics exercises is walking. Walking is not only a great cardio exercise but also an excellent way to lower stress. People walk for many reasons today: to free themselves of tensions, to find quiet.

You can do it outdoors or indoors on a treadmill. It will speed up your breath and your heart will beat faster, boosting your cardiovascular system, burning fat, and conditioning your body.

It is excellent because it will make you breathe harder, make your heart beat faster, improve your cardiovascular system, and at the same time, burning fat will condition your body.

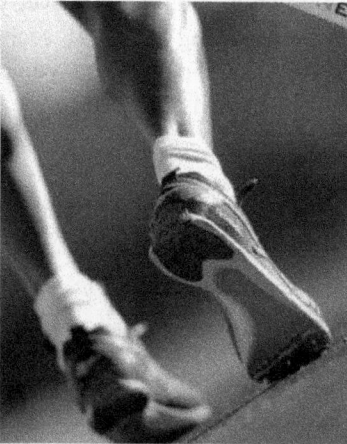

Walking is also a low-impact exercise, excellent for your knees and feet, and is almost injury-free. You don't need any equipment, and you can do it by yourself or with a partner.

The way I do it and is recommended by many experts is to walk fast for a couple of minutes, go slower for another couple of minutes, and then fast again. For 30 minutes, three or four times a week is plenty.

The benefits of walking are:

1. Cardiopulmonary fitness
2-Improve pulmonary function
3-Reduce body fat
4-More powerful leg

Walking is a low-impact exercise that is excellent for your knees and feet. Walking is a very popular activity. It is low cost, and you can change the intensity when you need to. This is a low-impact exercise because one foot is always in contact with the ground. You only need appropriate shoes. Your arms should swing in opposition to your legs.

Walking improves your heart and lungs and burns calories. When you increase your speed, you burn more calories.

If you increase your speed, your arm actions will increase too, and they will move in opposition to your legs. Being outside will help you feel calm and peaceful.

Walking is commonly injury-free and is as good as running or riding a bike. You can do it with friends or by yourself. The best way to do it is to walk fast for a couple of minutes, then go slower for another couple of minutes, and then fast again. Do it for 30 minutes, three or four times a week.

Walking benefits are:

Cardiovascular fitness   • Improved lung capacity
Reduce body fat   • Well-built legs

Want to look great in your "skinny jeans" or at the volleyball game at the beach with your friends but every diet you've tried has failed? Try walking.

Walking is the most effective way to shape your rear, lose fat at the waist, develop toned calves, and get slimmer thighs. It costs nothing, is easy. All you need is a good pair of shoes; no special gym or equipment is required. Best of all, speed-walking burns almost as many calories as jogging, but without damaging your joints.

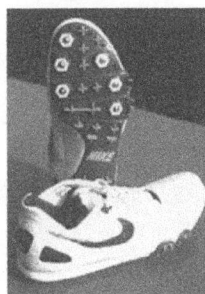

Laughter is inner jogging

WALK TIPS:

Good form

Walk tall, relax your shoulders, and bend your elbows at 90-degree angles. Land on your heels and roll through your feet, pushing off firmly with your toes for maximum calf-toning benefit.

Alternate speeds.

Begin slowly and gradually increase your pace to a brisk walk; alternate between fast and slow walking for two minutes and one minute.

Going uphill

If you add a climb to your walk, you will increase the number of calories burned, and it will also help tone your rear and legs too.

Walk up the stairs at a park or stadium bleachers, or in a hilly location in your local park.

If you're exercising on a treadmill, select the walking option with an incline.

Daily walks should be included.

Walking

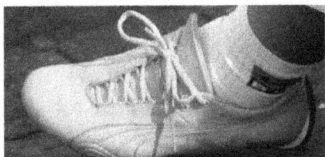

Every female would like to look great in jeans and in a bikini at the beach, right? Every single man wants to look great at the beach, at work or on a picnic, right? And you're gaining nothing from your gym workouts. Are you also tired of trying all those popular diets? What should you do?

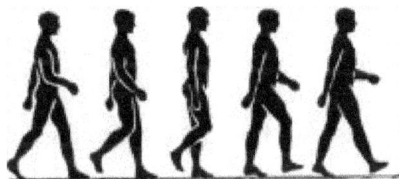

I'm repeating myself, but walking is the most efficient way to shape your buttocks. It also helps you develop and tone your calves, and it will get you results. Your thighs will be slimmer. It is free, it is easy, and no one has to teach you to do it. All you need is a good pair of shoes; no equipment is necessary.

Speed-walking burns almost as many calories as jogging, but it is much better for your joints. Walking is a great stress reliever and anyone can do it; the old, the young, the middle-aged, the elderly, women, men, and athletes.

Walking is an incredible exercise and will help you tone up, lose weight, and get into great shape. Start slowly; it took you years to get out of shape.

Increase the distance and time every week. It doesn't take long. Just walk fast for a couple of minutes, then slow down for a few.

That is all. It is especially good early in the morning with an empty stomach. I'm proof of this and a true believer in the early concept.

The University of Colorado researchers at Boulder declared good news for walkers: when overweight people stroll, they burn more calories per mile than brisk walking does, which also helps them reduce the risk of arthritis and injuries to the joints than walking alone.

They determined that obese people burned more calories by walking at a slower pace for a longer time than by walking at a faster speed.

A brisk walk is good for the brain.

Walking will enhance your memory and make you think faster. The benefits of walking are proven, and most people, by now, know about walking. A daily dose of 30 minutes of brisk walking is great for your heart, lungs, muscles, blood pressure, and bones.

Now we find out it's also good for your brain.

Research at the University of Pittsburgh shows that walking a few miles per week can postpone the progression of Alzheimer's disease. University research reveals that people who walk a minimum of 5 miles a week have bigger brains, enhanced memories, and mental ability in contrast to those who do not walk.

In another study led by Dr. Arthur F. Kramer, researchers from the University of Illinois at Urbana-Champaign indicated that walking builds muscles and also builds connectivity between brain paths.

This is significant because as we grow older, the connectivity between those circuits decreases and alters how well we do everyday tasks, such as driving.

The study: For one year, Kramer's team monitored 70 adults, from 60 to over 80 years old. All of them were inactive previously when the study began. The members were divided into two groups. One performed aerobic walking; the others did toning, stretching, and strengthening exercises.

The outcomes: Those who walked briskly reaped the biggest benefits--and not just physically, Kramer writes in the journal *Frontiers in Aging Neuroscience.* As the older people became more fit, the aerobic exercise actually improved their memory, attention, and several other cognitive processes.

In fact, the coherence among different regions in the brain networks increased so much that it actually mimicked that of the 20-somethings.It took a full year of walking for the consequences to be noticed. The six-month test results revealed no important brain differences. The individual that did stretching and strengthening exercises only noticed no cognitive benefit.

Another study reached the same conclusion. A recent study from the Harvard School of Public Health tracked more than 18,000 women ages 70 to 81 and determined that the more active we are the superior our cognition is. Certainly, walking one-and-a-half hours a week at a pace of one mile every 16–20 minutes produces the full cognitive benefits.

The National Center for Health Statistics said that about 60 million Americans are considered obese. Overweight adults are more at risk for knee osteoarthritis, which can cause painful stiffness.

Take the stairs at work instead of the elevator, or leave your desk for a brisk lunchtime walk around the building. Run errands on foot instead of driving.

"Walking is the best possible exercise habituate yourself to walk very far"
Thomas Jefferson

The Feet

Let's not forget the feet. Every time I have looked at a muscle/health magazine or book, I have been surprised that almost none of them talk about the feet. You are probably saying, "Why the hell the feet?" Think about it. Without good feet, we can't jog, run, or do cardiovascular exercises. Feet are abused every day, especially by women wearing high heels.

The athlete's body is like a race car; everything must be working in perfect, top-notch condition. You will walk an estimated 100,000 miles over the course of your life.

Some problems related to these are: Achilles Tendonitis, Callus, ingrown nails, shin splints, and Plantar Fasciitis, the most painful and bothersome being the infamous heel spurs.

That's why you should take care of your feet and always wear good exercise shoes. If you have diabetes, you must check your feet every day. This is a must.

Bones: Each foot contains 26 bones.
Joints: There are more than 30 joints in each foot.
Muscle-contracting and relaxing muscles help your feet move.
Tendons: The largest tendon in your foot is the Achilles.

Examples:
Plantar Fasciitis is characterized by a stabbing pain at the bottom of your foot, near the heel.

Achilles tendinitis: pain in the back of your lower leg or above your heel.

Stress fracture: tenderness and pain in a bony area of your foot.

Fitness-Cardio

Aerobics is a sustained movement that makes you use oxygen as fuel, like running, swimming, etc. Anaerobic exercise is quick, intense exercise like lifting weights, isometrics, etc.

Activities that are fast and short help you gain cardiovascular endurance and burn calories, such as walking, running, swimming, and cycling.

This way, you burn glucose and fat as fuel. So keep this in mind next time you hit the gym.

I know many people don't like to do aerobics, but you will continue to burn fat for hours after you stop exercising, even at rest.

This is great. Don't you think so?

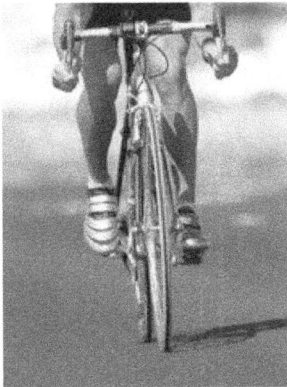

Now you don't have any excuse not to do your cardiovascular exercises or listen to music when using the treadmill or the stationary bicycle. Just do it.

These are types of fitness:

Aerobic Capacity
Agility balance
Flexibility
Power Speed

Cycling outside or inside is an excellent cardio exercise.

How often?

Three or two days a week, depending on how tough your cardiovascular exercise was last time, your health, your goals, and how fast you recuperated from your last workout.

How much?

Intensity depends on your age, weight, and goals. How long? If you really worked hard, fifteen to twenty-five minutes is about right.

How to progress?

The plan is to never allow your body to get used to the exercise, which is why I recommend altering the exercise time, reps, weight, and tempo.

Never do the same exercises twice in a row. Change and surprise your muscles. This way, your body will always react to your training, but it is also much safer to avoid tennis elbows and injuries.

If you are doing the same workouts over and over, you need to change exercises, weight, or tempo if you want to make progress.

The human body adapts fast and stops progressing, and when this happens, you don't improve anymore.

Long Workout

People believe that longer workouts equal better or faster results. Not true, intensity does.

"Insanity: doing the same thing over and over again and expecting different results".

Albert Einstein

Cardio Exercises

Treadmills—every gym has one. I would suggest walking fast for 2 minutes and then slowly for another 2 minutes, alternating for 30 minutes, 2 or 3 times a week. A treadmill is much better for your knees than running or jogging on the pavement. **The treadmill** is the most popular equipment in the gym. This is a great way to improve cardiovascular health. You can walk, jog, or run in place. You can increase the intensity by running faster, using an incline or decline. The best thing is to lessen the impact of walking or running on concreate, because the treadmill platform is flexible and has higher shock absorption than outdoors.

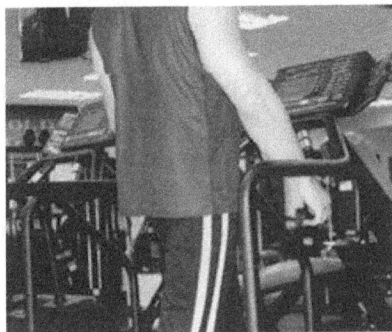

You are using the quadriceps, hamstrings, gluteal and gastrocnemius (the calf muscles), anterior tibialis (shin muscle) and the ankle joints. In the gym, you don't have to worry about weather, traffic, or dogs.

Cycling is excellent for people with back problems because it places less stress on your feet and ankles. It is excellent as a conditioning exercise because it will build the quadriceps (front of the thighs). Do it for about 30 minutes.3 times a week.

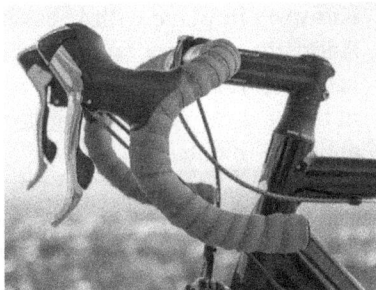

Cycling is an excellent cardiovascular exercise that reduces heart disease, high blood pressure, and burns calories, while also strengthening the quadriceps and hamstrings. Cycling has become an alternative to motorized transportation and is much more efficient than walking. Cycling outside is a great way to observe the scenery and is a great stress reliever. Cycling is a non-impact activity and an alternative to running.

Safety must be considered. Prevention is important. A good helmet is recommended to avoid injuries, and if you are going to ride at night, you should also wear reflective clothes.

Stair climbing is an outstanding conditioning exercise, great for your heart, lungs, and fat-loss. You will get into shape very quickly. Go up and down the stairs, increasing the time as you get in better shape.

Stair steppers: one of the most popular pieces of gym equipment for aerobic workouts; you use the quadriceps, hamstrings, gastrocnemius, anterior tibiae, and ankle joints. This is a non-impact exercise.

It is a fantastic cardiovascular exercise and will increase muscular strength.

Skip rope is an excellent conditioning exercise . It is beneficial to your lungs, heart, and fat loss, as well as to the development of your legs and calves. Alternate from foot to foot and do about 55 jumps per minute. Don't do it on a hard surface. It can hurt your shins if you do it on a hard surface. Always wear proper footwear. Jump for two or three minutes, alternating fast and slow, stop for a minute, repeat again. Personally, this is one of my favorite cardio exercises. Excellent conditioning exercise. Four times a week for 15 min.

Running in place with knees high is very good cardio exercise. Another one of my favorites, because you don't need any equipment, just raise your knees high. You may raise your feet higher as you get in better shape. Excellent indoor exercise. Three times a week for about 15 minutes.

Jogging conditions your heart, plus all the benefits of walking. This is a high-impact exercise that places some strain on the body, the muscles, and especially the joints of the knees.

While jogging, you should transfer your weight evenly from one foot to the other. Again, good specific shoes should be worn. Jogging is much more efficient than walking.

Running is very popular in many parts of the world. People run for many reasons. Some do it to lose weight; others do it for their heart and lung health. Many runners often experience a release of endorphins, commonly referred to as "runner high." This feeling acts as a catalyst for weight loss, stress relief and a sense of well-being, not only physically but also mentally.

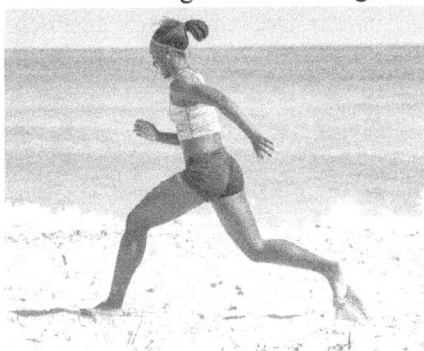

Running burns more calories than jogging because you consume more oxygen. It is also a high-impact exercise, which can lead to more joint injuries.

You can increase the intensity by running on an incline hill or on a downhill terrain. For safety reasons, the surfaces should be taken into consideration. It is better to run on a softer surface like grass instead of pavement or concrete to reduce the risk of injuries to your knees, shins, ankles, and low back.

Sprint go slowly at first, keeping your breathing steady and rhythmic, with a peak at a higher intensity followed by active recovery. Sprinting will make you muscular, obtain definition, and make you lean like a race horse. This is one of the best exercises to get in top shape, but make no mistake; it is also a very tough exercise to do. Many champions, including top bodybuilders, use it.

You run really fast to your marking point, then you return to your starting point. You don't return to rest, instead you walk back slowly, breathing to regain your breathing back to normal, as your active recovery, then you sprint again. This is an excellent way to burn calories, lose weight, and get in shape. You have to start sprinting slowly, warm up, and make sure you have your doctor's clearance. Work yourself up, little by little.

The sprint and recovery intervals let you train at a higher intensity. This kind of exercise should only be done three times per week because it is a hard exercise.

If you are overweight, stationary bicycles are ideal. You can adjust the tension to your needs. High tension is used to build thigh muscles. Tension down for a cardiovascular workout. Go fast, slow down, and alternate. Three to four times a week for 30 min. You are using the quadriceps, hamstrings, gastrocnemius, anterior tibiae, and ankle joints. This is a non-impact exercise; you don't have to worry about the weather. Modern stationary bikes are smaller, sleeker, and better looking than outdoor bikes.

Rowing Machine - This is a fantastic aerobic exercise. Another favorite of mine, great aerobic exercise.

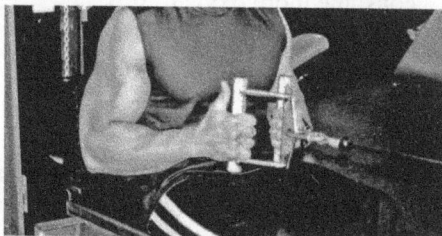

Excellent for the arms, back, and legs while you get cardiovascular benefits at the same time. Four times a week for about 20 minutes. Rowing machines simulate rowing a boat, which is a great exercise. It is a great exercise that will give you a good upper and lower body workout and, at the same time, give you an excellent cardiovascular workout. It is low-impact, so it causes fewer joint problems.

It involves the gluteus maximus, the quadriceps, the hamstrings, and the muscles of the lower legs. The upper body includes the back muscles, the trapezius and rhomboids, the biceps, and the triceps. If you set the resistance high, you are working harder and developing muscles. If you only want aerobics, you should set the resistance at a lower setting. Rowing is a great cardiovascular exercise that strengthens the upper body and the lower body at the same time. One of my favorite pieces of equipment!

Swimming is a popular and often recommended exercise among doctors and therapists. Excellent aerobic exercise. Keep in mind that some experts think it does not decrease body fat. This you have to discover for yourself. Do it three times a week for 30 minutes. For safety reasons, don't swim alone. Swimming is a great exercise that works the whole body and increases your cardiovascular endurance. Swimming is not always convenient.

You have to have a pool in your home. You use muscles like the gluteal, hamstrings, quadriceps, and the upper body muscles as well. These include the deltoids, Latissimus Dorsi, Trapezius, the biceps, and triceps.

Here is a controversy. Many famous bodybuilders and experts claim that as a result of being in the water, the body reacts by keeping fat to keep warm, making you fat. Swimming is considered to have a low risk of injuries, but it carries some risks. Here are some of them.

Exposure to chemicals: chlorine and chlorine inhalation
Diving into a submerged object at the bottom of the pool
Drowning-never practice alone, swim supervised by lifeguards.
If you are careful, you can avoid some of these situations. This is a popular form of exercise. I don't have any experience with it; I'm listing it here for information.

Jumping Jacks – How can anyone forget this exercise from gym class in elementary school? Better to practice on the grass to make it less traumatic on your heels and knees. Do about 30 reps, increasing reps as you get in shape, four times a week.

Dancing: As a matter of fact, Sergio Oliva the Myth, multiples Bodybuilding Championship winner, used to go dancing all the time and he would go dancing the night before a major competition. He believed that because of his dancing, he was always in good cardiovascular shape.

Plyometric- Many athletes from different sports use this system to get into shape. Training with exercises that use speed and force of different exercises to build muscle and power.

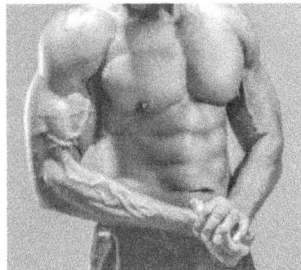

Warm up-Do 10 to 20 jumping jacks, move around, lift your knees a couple of time, swing your body. Warm up depends in you physical level and I believe in age.

We seal our fate with the choices we make.
Gloria Estefan

Fitness

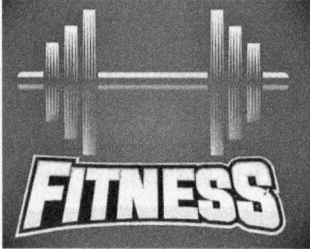

Aerobics is a sustained movement that makes you use oxygen as fuel, like running, swimming, etc. Anaerobic exercise is quick, intense exercise like lifting weights, isometrics, etc. Activities that are fast and short help you gain cardiovascular endurance and burn calories.

Such as walking, running, swimming, and cycling. This way, you burn glucose and fat as fuel. So keep this in mind next time you hit the gym. I know many people don't like to do aerobics, but you will continue to burn fat for hours after you stop exercising, even at rest. This is great. Don't you think so?

Now you don't have any excuse not to do your cardiovascular exercises or listen to music when using the treadmill or the stationary bicycle. Just do it. Keep in mind that jogging is a high-impact exercise that puts strain on your body's joints, mostly in the joints of the knee. Some people can develop pain in their lower back and hips.

There are six types of fitness, including:

Strength	Flexibility
Aerobic Capacity	Power
Agility and balance	Speed

Aerobics Best

1. Jogging	6. Dancing
2. Cycling	7. Stair Climbing
3. Skip-Rope	8. Walking
4. Tennis	9. Weight-Training
5. Rowing	10. Sprinting

90

High-speed cardio routine to burn off flab

I see people in the gym using the cardio machine for a very long time, sometimes for an hour, at a slow or medium pace. I know for a fact that this is not the way to go.

I weigh the same as I did in high school: 175 pounds. Quicker results can be achieved with a short cardio workout.

When you do cardio fast and for short intervals, you can speed up your metabolism to burn calories for hours, even when you are sleeping later on. Intense and brief exercises have been proven to improve your cardio-vascular fitness and help you lose fat faster, period.

Caffeine in most parts of the world is legalized. Some research reveals that a small amount of caffeine can help burn fat before cardiovascular exercise, making the body more energetic by arousing the central nervous system. Too much caffeine can overwork the kidneys, lead to insomnia, and make you restless. Try my circuit. You can do it anywhere. As you progress, try to do it faster or take a shorter break in between.

How often should you do cardio?

It depends. How you respond, how much time you have to do cardio, how fast you want to lose weight, etc. Everybody is different. Time doing cardio for me may not be good for you, and this is something you have to find out for yourself.

When is a good time to do cardio?

I've always done it first thing in the morning; again, this is something you should figure out: work hours, school hours, and pick-up times for your children. Some scientific studies show that the body stores low glycogen after an overnight fast, and that the body will burn fat for energy.

Warm up

It is very important to warm up, do 10 to 20 jumping jacks, move around, lift your knees a couple of times, and swing your body. The idea is to get your heart and lungs ready for the coming workout. Rest only when moving to the next circuit. Rest and go to the next circuit.

As you advance, try to make your rest periods shorter until you can do all three circuits without stopping.

When you can do three or four circuits very fast without stopping, you will have amazing cardio-vascular fitness and, I'm sure, a very trim muscular body.

Circuit A
A- Body weight squat- Squat down parallel to the floor. Don't go down all the way. Do 25 reps

B- Knees high – Bring your knees as high as you can, alternate left and right, one rep is when both knees went up. Do 25 reps.

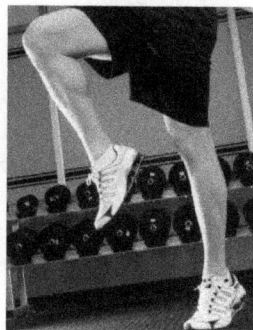

Knees high

C-Jumping Jack's Splint leap Instead of bringing your legs sideways, one leg goes to the front and the other to the back. Do 25 reps.

D-Body-weight jump: Jump high, land with your knees bent, squat down, and jump again without hesitating. Do 25 reps.

Circuit B

A-With a medicine ball, dumbbell or a heavy book, bend your knees, lower your body and swing the medicine ball/dumbbell between your legs. Bring it up to your chest high and keep swinging it up and down. Do 25 reps.

B-Back Legs-Squat trusts I'm sure you remember this one from school. I do.

Standing lower your body to a squat, place your hands on the floor in front of you like in a push-up position, and kick both your legs back at the same time. Fast brings your legs back to a squat, then stand up. Do 25 reps.

C- Jumping Jacks' Splint jump. Instead of bringing your legs sideways, one leg goes to the front and the other to the back. Do 25 reps.

Circuit C

A- Jump high, land with your knees bent and squat down, then jump again without pause. Up and down. Do 25 reps.

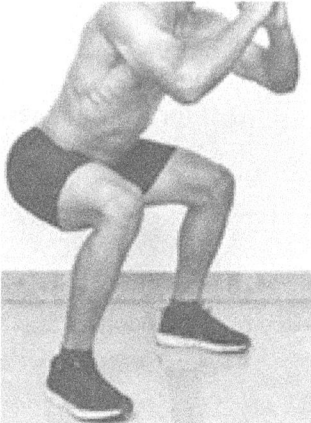

B-Fast Push-ups- From the push-up position lower your body; bend your elbows until chest almost touches the floor. Press yourself up very fast. Do 10 reps as fast as you can.

C-Jumping Jacks- I'm sure you also remember this one from school. Jump and spread your legs while clipping your hand in top of your head. Hands clasped in front of the chest are a variation. Do 25 reps. believe me when I say that after a few weeks, you will be surprised with your progress. Everybody is going to be asking you what your secret is. Now you know what short and intense circuit exercises are.

"The future depends on what you do today."
Mahatma Gandhi

Step Aerobics Cardio

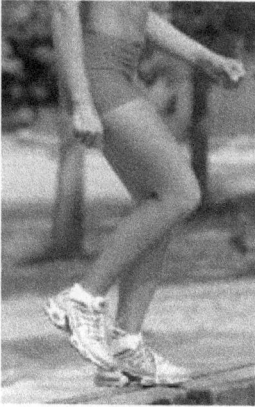

Numerous people do Step Aerobics each year. It is excellent, as good as running, but it's much safer and easier on your joints. Step Aerobics is the perfect workout to do at home. You can do it anywhere: in an apartment building, the living room, or stairs.

Stepping up and down stairs or blocks is an excellent cardio workout; you don't need any special equipment. It is a basic and simple training exercise. Have you tried going up and down the stairs? Believe me, it will get you in shape real fast.

Aerobic activity right after a demanding muscle-building workout would delay our response to the body's needs for nutrition, rest, and recuperation.

So... aerobics on off days works best.

I'm a hard gainer. I love weight training and have been doing it since 1962, and I had to discover the best way to train, the hard way.

Don't use extended workouts.

Brief, hard, heavy training

Follow a balanced diet

Get enough sleep and rest.

The idea is to increase poundage, short rest, less frequent training, more reps, low reps, vary the exercises, and change routines.

Men Calisthenics

The callisthenic circuit is something you can do anywhere. There are no weights or equipment; you can do it anywhere, anytime; your home, living room, backyard, beach, or a nearby park. This is an excellent, great cardiovascular workout that will also stimulate plenty of muscles.

Do each exercise for 20 seconds before going onto the next one.

Jumping jacks	Push-ups
Prisoner Squats	Jump rope (rope is optional).
High knees in place.	Push-ups
Power strides	Leg raises while standing.
Burpees	

Perform each sequence four to five times with no rest. You may think it is simple, but the truth is that this routine at the end will leave you completely gasping for air and exhausted.

Jumping Jacks

Standing position, with your feet shoulder width apart, with your arms down at your sides. At the same time, jump outward into a wide stance and bring your arms up overhead. Never land with locked knees. Return to the start in a smooth motion and repeat without pausing.

Prisoner Squats

Start in a standing position. Jump out of a squat and sink down into a squat. Keep your knees in line with your toes and avoid sticking out forward. Burst out into a jump, allowing the feet to leave the floor. Perform each sequence four to five times with no rest. You may think it is simple, but the truth is that this routine at the end will leave you completely gasping for air and exhausted.

High Knees

This exercise is like a version of jogging in place. You lift your knees high in a constant motion and alternate legs in a running motion, raising the knees high in this fashion each time.

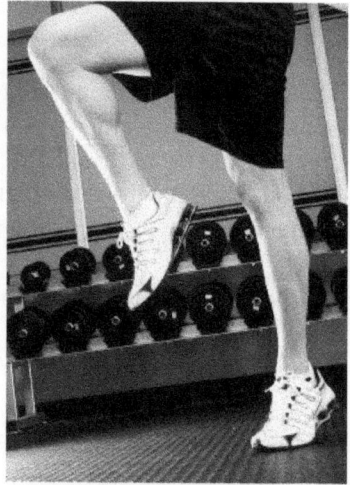

Power Strides

Power strides resemble speed skates. Instead of moving yourself back and forth, you move yourself each time in the same direction, landing on the same leg five times before changing direction, and doing the same with your other leg. It is done fast.

Burpees

Star in a standing position, go into a crouch position, and kick your legs back into a pushup position.

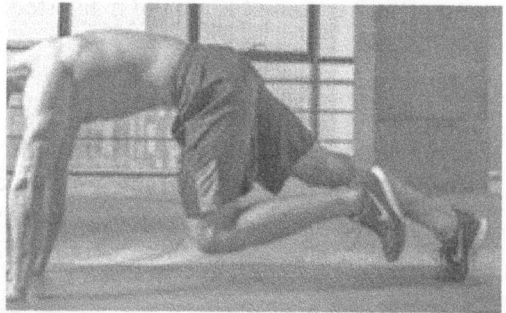

Jump the legs back into a crouch, and burst up into the air into a jump, allowing the feet to leave the ground. When you land, come back into a crouch position and repeat the movement without pausing.

"Life is like a riding bicycle. To keep balance, you must keep moving."
Albert Einstein

Women's Calisthenics Workout

Warm-up

You can do jumping jacks, run in place, or do dumbbell swings.

1-Dumbbell swing

With a dumbbell between your legs, hold it with two hands and swing it up and down for 8 or 10 reps.

Excellent warmup.

2-Stretched leg kick

Hips and thighs

Face down on the bench, lift one leg with the toe pointing backward as high as you can do, 8 or 10 reps.

3-Straight leg kicks to the side

Thighs and hips

Lying on your side Raise your leg to the side as far as you can, toes pointing upward. Do 8 or 10 reps each side.

4-Leg raise on the bench

Lower tummy

Flat on a bench, only to about the hips. Hold the sides of the bench and raise your legs until they are straight up.

Keep the tension on the abdominal muscles, going up and down for 8 or 10 reps.

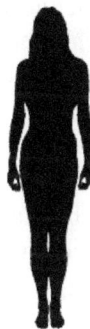

5-kneeling kicks in the back

Hips, waist & lower back

Get down on four, pick one knee and draw it forward toward your chin, bringing your head down as if they were going to meet, then extend the same leg backward and, at the same time, lift your head.

Repeat with each leg for 8 or 10 reps.

These are not only good warm-ups but also good exercises for the abdomen and legs.

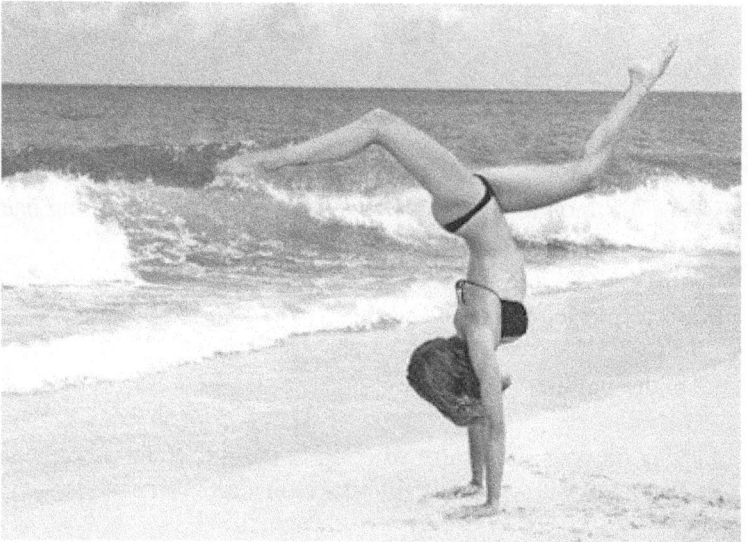

Free Exercise

You have to believe in yourself when no one else does.
Serena Williams

Stretching

Stretching should be a part of an exercise program. Stretching exercises are now commonly performed by coaches in a variety of sports, athletes, and dance instructors. Stretching, I believe, is very important to weight training; you can do it as a warm-up or on its own. Stretching after a warm-up prepares muscles for exercise. When muscles are warm, they are more flexible.

There are many good stretching exercises that must be done after the muscles are warmed up, never cold. Remember to spend most of your time building muscles. Don't overdo it. Be cautious. Stretch a little beyond your safety zone, but do not push through pain. Never stretch a cold muscle and make sure you are in the correct position. Never bounce during your stretch. Inhale deeply into the stretch and exhale when you release. Stretch for 15 minutes at least three times per week. Stop right away if you feel pain.

1st Leg Lift

Stand erect, lift your leg, and hold it straight in front of you. Hold your leg for a count of three. Do both legs 5 times each.

2-Leg curl
Stand a foot away from a wall. Keep your body straight and lean forward. Keep the heel on the floor, bend your leg backward, and pull your foot until you feel the stretch in your leg.

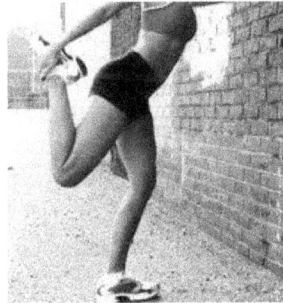

3-Circles
Standing erect, hold your arms straight out as if you were to fly. Rotate your arms slowly in a circle, backwards first then forwards. Do 10 in one direction, then 10 more the other.

4 -Neck Rotation
Standing erect, rotate your head slowly one way, then the other way. Do 10 reps each way.

5 Walks

Sitting on a stool or chair, walk with your hands between your knees.
You should try to place your hands flat on the floor, stretch them a
bit, and hold count for 10 seconds. Don't bounce, do 10 reps each
time, trying to go a little farther. Go slowly at first.

6: Pull up

Bend forward like you are touching your toes; grab each ankle with
both hands, pull up for a few seconds, release, and do 10 reps.

7-Side Bends

Standing straight Raise your left arm high and place your other hand
against your right leg. Stretch upward as high as you can with your
left hand while you bend your body to the right. Alternate left and
right. Repeat 10 times.

8-Thigh Stretches

Lay face down on the floor, bend your knees, and grasp your knees
with your hand and hold them for 30 seconds. Release and repeat 5
times with both knees.

9 – Calves' stretch
Stand a foot away from a wall. Keep your body straight and lean
forward. Keep the heel
on the floor until you
feel the stretch in your
calves.
 Repeat 5 times.

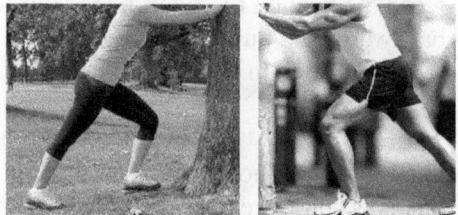

10 -Triceps Stretches
With arms over head, gently pull one elbow behind your head and
hold the stretch for a few seconds with the other hand.
Switch arms, repeat 5 times each.

Stretching is a must for both men and women

Interval Training

This is my favorite training for getting and staying in shape and exercising to burn fat. For years, it was impossible for me to lose my spare tire. If I diet, I get too skinny. In my 55 years of training, this is the best method I have found to get in shape. Interchanged with my other routines, it is amazing the results I got, and you can also get them in just 15 minutes. I do this early in the morning with almost an empty stomach, just a small cup of coffee and water. This makes my body use body fat for energy. Then, and only then, I do have breakfast. Most of the time, like an hour or two after I finish exercising. It makes me feel great for the rest of the day.

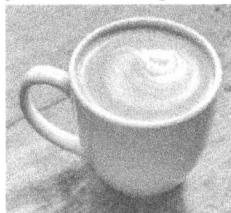

Interval training- HIT is a brief, intense burst of aerobic exercise (fast walking, running, or biking). The combination of fast and slow training has improved my cardiovascular and fitness level and kept me in shape and toned at the same weight I used to weigh in high school.

Make sure to always warm up correctly. This is very important, especially if you are older or overweight. Take 5 minutes to warm up. Swing your arms around, do 10 jumping jacks, dance a little bit, and walk fast. I don't believe in stretching before exercise, only after I'm done training.

The intensity should be based on your fitness level. Use common sense. Try walking fast for a few days and see how you feel. Get into shape slowly. It took you years to get out of shape. Determination, discipline, and perseverance are what make warriors.

Your goal should be to develop a balanced and symmetrical body; an imbalance in muscle development will cause chronic pain and some disability later in life. Working your arms and chest, for example, will give you rotator cuff trouble later on as a result of the imbalanced muscles, and if you have weak abdominal development because you never work the abdominal muscles, you will definitely develop lower back trouble years later.

Jumping Rope

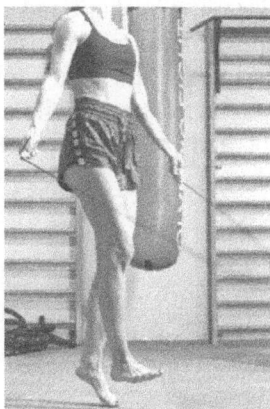

Jump rope is a fun way to exercise. It is one of the best aerobic workouts because it works the whole body, develops coordination, enhances speed and muscular strength, and is excellent for the heart, lungs, circulation, as well for your waist line. The correct way to find out the appropriate rope side is to step on the center of the rope and pull. Keep the handles up; they must be near to the middle of your chest.

Suggestions:

Wear shoes with a cushioned ball of the foot. Aerobics or cross-training shoes are the best for jumping rope. Use a mat, a gym floor or a wood floor. Try not to do it on concrete, which is the worst for your feet. Keep your head up and your back straight. Don't jump high, just low enough to pass the rope under your feet.

Basic moves:

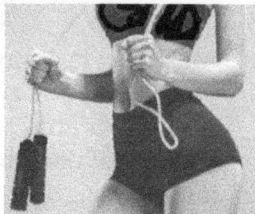

Double Bounce: Jump two times with both feet in one rotation of the rope.

Alternate foot: both feet alternated up and down while the rope rotates

High Knee: bring your knees very high with each jump.

Scissors: Legs back and forth, one leg to the front, one back in a motion, alternate right foot front, and left foot in front. Try to jump gently.

Toe tap: Touch your toes on the floor in front of you and tap them

If you don't have a rope, just go through the motions with an imaginary rope. You still get a great workout. My favorite.

Cross steps: while you are in the air during the jump movement, you land with your legs crossed.

Excellent practice. That's why boxers use the rope to get in shape.

Running steps: a slightly faster jog pace to increase the intensity.

You only need ten minutes a day. Just give it a shot. Maybe you'll like it as much as I do!

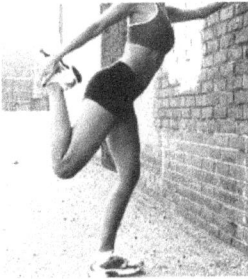

Stretching-The object of stretching exercises is to keep flexible and increase your range of motion.

Don't bounce; bouncing makes the muscles contract. You don't want this when stretching; this is the opposite of what you are aiming for.

We know the significance of stretching in bodybuilding. Start slowly.

Rest time: Keep the workout as fast as possible, but without giving up performance. The real idea is to rest for the smallest total time required to recuperate for the next set. Your level of fitness must determine how long or short you should rest. Never go by a clock or count time during rest periods.

Do as I do, take a few steps, walk around breathing. As soon as you can breathe more normally go back to your next set. Make your breathing or the need for air your guide.

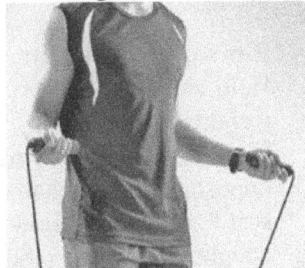

Mood benefits

Exercises lift your mood, no question about it. Runners talk about a high, usually known as "runner's high." This is the release of endorphins through exercise, and the blood flowing to the brain then produces a sense of wellbeing. It also lowers the stress. Many people exercise or run looking for this feeling.

30-minutes fast circuit workout

This 30-minute circuit workout is great if your time is tight. You only need a set of 5- to 8-pound dumbbells. Warm up by walking or light jogging for three minutes. You'll rotate through the cardiovascular and strength movements described here, completing the entire circuit twice. At the end, cool down and do some stretching at the end of the circuit. You could add abdominal work at the end if you wish.

Cardio Shuffles: With feet spread wide, shuffle sideways back and forth across the floor for one minute. No rest-move to the next exercise.

Push-ups (for the chest): Lower your body until your chest is about a fist's distance from the floor; push up until arms are fully extended. Do eight to 12 repetitions. No rest-move to next exercise.

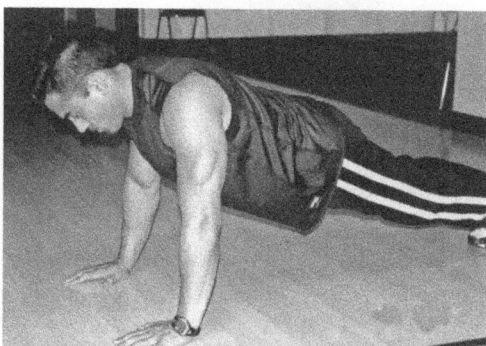

Cardio Jumping Jacks: Perform a minute of jumping jacks. No rest-move to next exercise.

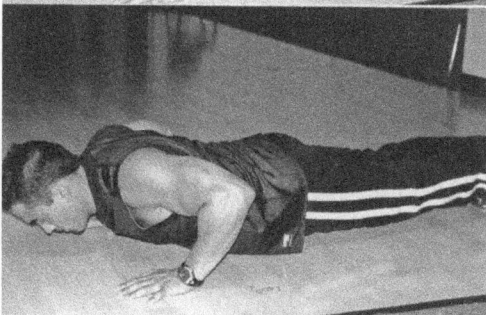

Rows (for the back): Hold one dumbbell weights in one hand; bend at the hips, placing opposite hand on chair seat for support. Allow the arm to extend toward the floor with the weight. Bend your elbow as you pull your arm back. The elbows should point toward the ceiling; the weights should end up right at the waistline. Release it slowly toward the floor. Repeat eight to twelve times on the opposite side. No rest-move to the next exercise.

Cardio ski jumps: for one minute, jump side to side while keeping your feet together. No rest-move to the next exercise.

Rear Flyes (for the upper back): With a dumbbell in each hand, bend from the hips until the upper body is parallel with the floor. Lift weights up and back, leading with the elbows.

Concentrate on squeezing your shoulder blades together, as if you were pinching a small ball between them. Pause, release slowly, and repeat for a total of eight to 12 repetitions. No rest-move to the next exercise.

Jumping rope use a jumping rope or pretend to turn a rope while skipping or jogging for one minute; keep your arms flexed for a more vigorous workout. No rest-move to the next exercise.

Dips (for the triceps): Grip the edge of a chair or a table edge. Legs should be close together, knees bent, and toes pointed up. Slowly lower your bottoms, and then push up until your arms are straight. Straighten the legs slightly to intensify the exercise. Perform eight to 12 repetitions. No rest-move to the next exercise.

Cardio Jog: Jog in place with your knees high for one minute, making sure to keep your knees high. No rest-move to the next exercise.

Standing Curls (for the biceps): Stand straight with one weight in each hand, arms at your sides. Bend both arms at the elbow, slowly bringing the weights toward the shoulders. Keep your arms and elbows close to your body and lower them slowly. Perform eight to 12 repetitions.

When you can do the circuit three times, you are going to be in great shape.

"It is a sin not to do what one is capable of doing"
Jose Marti

Exercise-Men

A recent report indicates that men with higher cardiorespiratory fitness levels are many times less likely to acquire prostate cancer than men with low cardiorespiratory fitness levels.

A Study Shows That Building Muscle Extends Life.

A study conducted at UCLA showed that a man's life expectancy is prolonged by seven minutes for every minute spent exercising. The same study showed that older people who had more muscle mass were less likely to die of any disease than people of their own age with lower muscle mass.

When you begin training and you are young, anything works. No matter how or what you do, you grow. A few months later, as you progress, you need more training intensity. Soreness and stiffness are common and are a natural response to exercise. This goes away as you get used to the exercise.

Nothing is new or different. The answer is hard work. Routines haven't changed, and the exercises, sets, and reps haven't changed either.

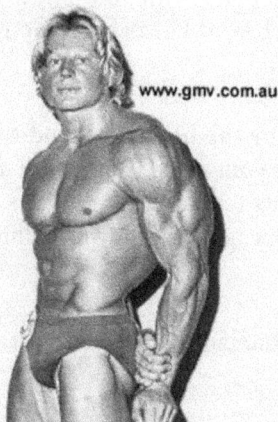

www.gmv.com.au

Dave Draper - The blond bomber-Mr. America-Mr. Universe
Photo courtesy Wayne Gallasch

"Attention to health is life's greatest hindrance"
Plato

106

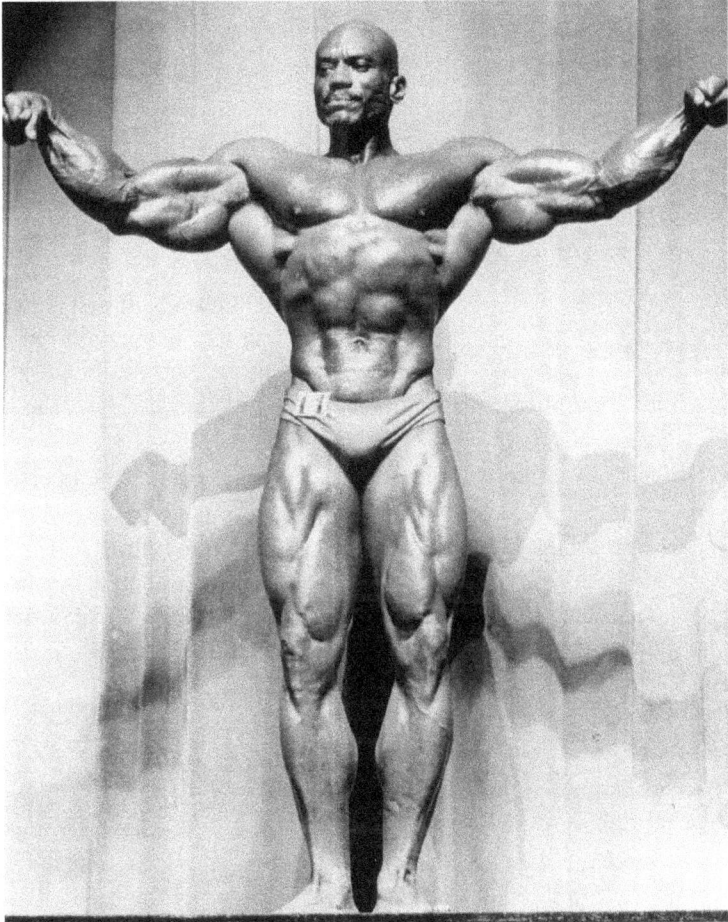

Sergio Oliva The Myth
Courtesy of R. Kennedy Musclemag

Mid-section

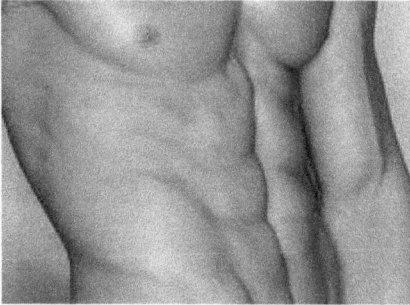

It's not the Diet!

The word diet originally comes from the Greek word "diaita," which means "manner of living."

Thousands of diets have been written in the past, but do all those diets really work? Think about it for a moment.

Six packs are the finishing touch for a lean, well-shaped person.

The first thing you see in a person is their midsection. A trim abdomen adds tremendous appeal to a person's body. The upper body appears much bigger and more muscular, and the whole body looks attractive to a man or a woman, it does not matter.

Drink water during your workouts.

Drink before and after exercising.

Eat three good meals a day. If you can handle it, eat 6 meals a day if you are trying to gain weight.

Don't miss a workout unless you are sick.

Get sufficient rest and sleep at least eight hours every night.

The abdominal muscles

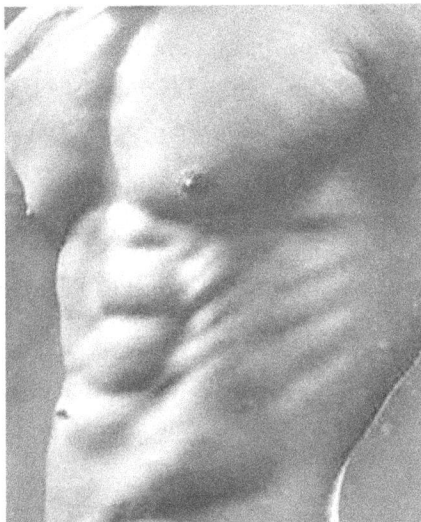

The abdominal muscle is extremely vital to your health. They are in the middle of your body and support every movement you make.

A trim, small waist or 6 packs naturally is very eye-catching and sexy. Also, the abdominal muscles are very important in reducing back pain and stabilizing the spine.

The belly fat of the obliques hounds me too. I had to get downright skinny to reduce it. There goes the muscle mass, energy, and power to produce muscle.

There is no way out. The only way to obtain an outstanding abdominal is to do aerobics with a wise low-fat, low-calorie diet.

That is it! No tricks, no secrets.

Crunch

One of the best exercises for the abdomen

Excellent exercise. See the abdomen section. Exhale as you go up and inhale as you go down. One of the exercises preferred by the exercise guru, Vince Gironda.

As I previously stated, I began reading the work of Vince Gironda, the most controversial bodybuilding trainer in the history of bodybuilding, as a competitor, instructor, and gym owner, in my early years. I learned a lot from Vince, just as I also learned a lot from Arthur Jones.

Drink water during your workouts. Drink before and after exercising. Eat three good meals a day. If you can handle it, eat 6 meals a day if you are trying to gain weight.

Don't miss a workout unless you are sick.
Get sufficient rest and sleep at least eight hours every night.

Breathing--It is very important to breathe correctly. Never hold your breath during the hardest part of an exercise or lift. Instead of exhaling,

Crunch -Exhale as you go up and inhale as you go down

Vince Gironda- He believed in kelp supplementation to increase your metabolic rate. Not synthetic iodine, but ocean kelp, which contains a good amount of nutrients. Kelp tablets are made from pure ocean kelp.

Eat three good meals a day. If you can, eat 6 meals a day if you are trying to gain weight. You must drink water during your workouts. Drink before and after exercising.

Don't miss a workout unless you are sick. Get sufficient rest and sleep at least eight hours every night.

Core Training

According to the American Dietetic Association, a waistline larger than 34 inches in women and 40 inches in men increases the risk of many health conditions, including heart disease and diabetes.

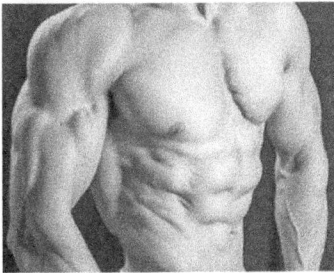

Your midsection

The abdominal muscles lie between the ribs and the pelvis at the front of the body. The abdominal muscles reinforce the torso, allow movement, and keep organs in position by regulating internal abdominal pressure. This includes the ab muscles on the front, the lower back muscles and glutes on the back, the diaphragm on the top, and the pelvic floor and hip muscles on the bottom.

Stress: If you have stress or job-related stress, cortisol levels remain high, and your body responds by placing extra fat on your abs. The abdomen is a major target for the stress hormone cortisol.

Mediterranean Diet: The Mediterranean diet has an anti-inflammatory effect. Olive oil, fatty fish, nuts, and seeds are good fats that influence the body. The omega-3 fats in those foods decrease the hormone called adrenaline, which results in less belly fat.

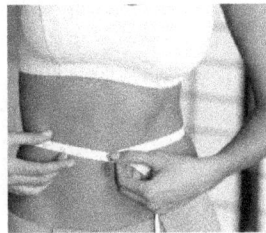

Better snack: A study from Pennsylvania State University found that eating 2-3 ounces per day of walnuts is great for a healthy diet, with positive changes in the gut.

Cardio: Do at least 15 to 30 minutes of heart-pumping cardio at least three days a week. Cardio really engages your whole body.

Mass training

Squats
The bench press
Bent-over Barbell Row
Standing barbell press
The Lat machine pulls
down
Barbell curls
Routines should be
changed frequently, and exercises so your body never adjusts.

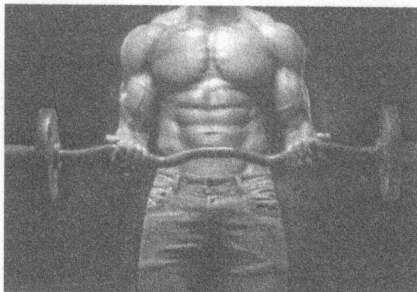

The Pyramid system
This is the system the great legend Sergio Oliva used. He did antagonist muscles, like working biceps and triceps.

Injury
It is no secret that when you grow older, it takes more time to recover and, at the same time, it is easier to get hurt or develop an injury.

Focus on safety.
Concentrate when working out. Always warm up and cool down. Never sit down after working out or doing exercise. Walk a little bit around if you need to get your breath back.

If something hurts, stop right away and do something else. Skip that exercise for a couple of days. If you are doing weight training, your first set should always be a light set. Don't use too heavy a weight. Be careful when doing squats. Do not drop down fast and do not bounce. This could damage your knees.

Better to train with a partner than alone. Sergio Oliva tells a story in his book, Sergio Oliva the Myth, Building the Ultimate Physique, that one time he was doing an extremely heavy bench press and he got stuck under the weight with no one around to help him. He had to roll the weight down from his body, which was very scary!

Don't rush into exercise after breaks, take your time.

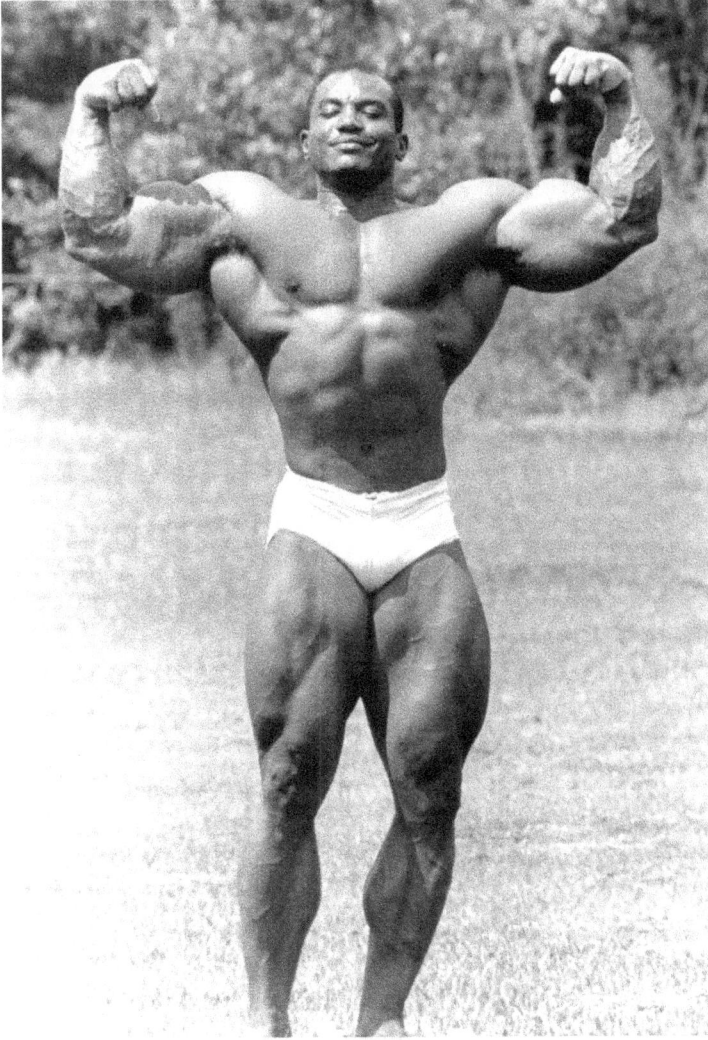

Sergio Oliva Deland Beach Fl,
Photo by Inge Cook-Jones Courtesy of Arthur Jones

Secret

Like Sergio Oliva said in his great book, Sergio Oliva the Myth-Building the Ultimate Physique. They are not secrets, but hard workouts.

Use heavy compound exercises.
Use correct repetitions.
Restorative time
Train cautiously.
You must increase resistance to add size. **At all times!**

Remember, an injury could take months to heal and you might have to stop training for months.

Tips to keep in mind:
For legs

The deadlift is not a back lift.
Don't try to jerk the weight.

<u>Best Exercises</u>

Chins	Deadlift
Dips	Dumbbell Row
Bent-over barbell row	Front Press
Lat Pulley to the front	Curls
T-bar row	Lateral Raises
Bench Press (better inclined)	Triceps pull down

Warm up
1-light set
1 medium set
1 heavy set

Exercises like the bent-over barbell and the T-bar can be very dangerous for your low back if you jerk the weight or if you are careless.

Strength training

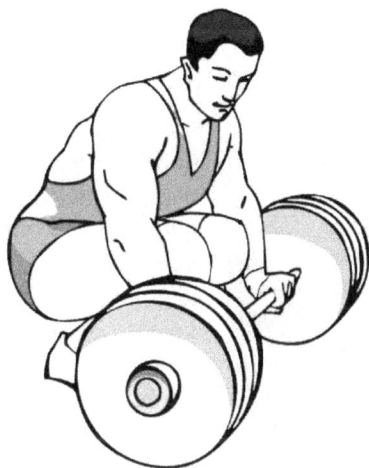

According to the American Council on Sports Medicine (ACSM) and the American Heart Association, everybody needs to include strength training twice a week as part of a fitness routine.

Research specifies that strength workouts are safe for all ages and that teaming up with aerobic exercise can enhance your physical and mental health.

Strength training is beneficial for older adults, but more for the reasons that slow the loss of bone and muscle that goes along with aging.

Other benefits include:

•Weight control
•Lowering the risk of type 2 diabetes
•Relief from arthritis
•Better balance and fall prevention
•Improved cardiovascular health
•Fighting depression

Strength training is usually divided into sets and repetitions. Repetitions, or "reps," are the number of times you do an exercise. A group of repetitions—usually between 8 and 15—is called a set.

If you are able to do more than one set of an exercise, add more. Always rest for a few minutes between sets. The ACSM recommends 8 to 10 strength training exercises of 8 to 10 repetitions each, twice a week

Strength Training Equipment Options

There is a wide range of strength-training equipment available. Here are the choices:

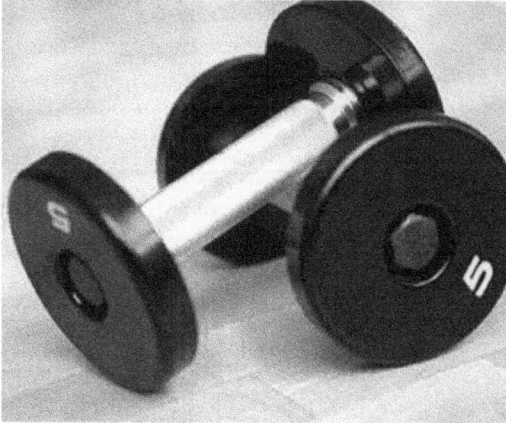

Free weights: Barbells are long bars with weights attached at the ends. Dumbbells are smaller, hand-held weights. The advantages of free weights are that they are inexpensive and handy.

Machines: Strength training with machines is as effective as free weights, plus machines have the advantage of being safer and easier to use.

Since strength training machines are designed to exercise specific muscle groups, you can get a faster, more efficient workout by moving from machine to machine. The disadvantage is that machines are not portable and can be expensive, so you may be limited to using exercise machines at a gym.

Stability balls: These strength-training gadgets look like overgrown, colorful beach balls, but can be very useful pieces of exercise equipment. By learning exercises that include body curves and rolls using different positions on the stability ball, you can strengthen the essential core muscles in your body. The benefit of the stability ball is that it is inexpensive and adaptable to many uses.

Weighted body bars: Body bars are foam-covered weights that may be used in a total body workout class to combine aerobic exercise with strength training. They are reasonably inexpensive.

Body bars are available in different weights to fit your strength and ability.

Disadvantage: Because they are about 4 feet long, they can be difficult to carry around, so they are not ideal for traveling with.

Exercise bands: Bands are portable and inexpensive. They are just big elastic bands with different degrees of tension, and as your strength increases, you will need to graduate to stronger sets of resistance bands.

Kettlebells: This tool was developed in Russia for use in strength training and aerobic exercise to work all muscle groups at the same time. It looks similar to a cannonball with a handle.

A kettlebell workout is high-intensity and involves a full range of motion. It requires the ability to stretch and be flexible.

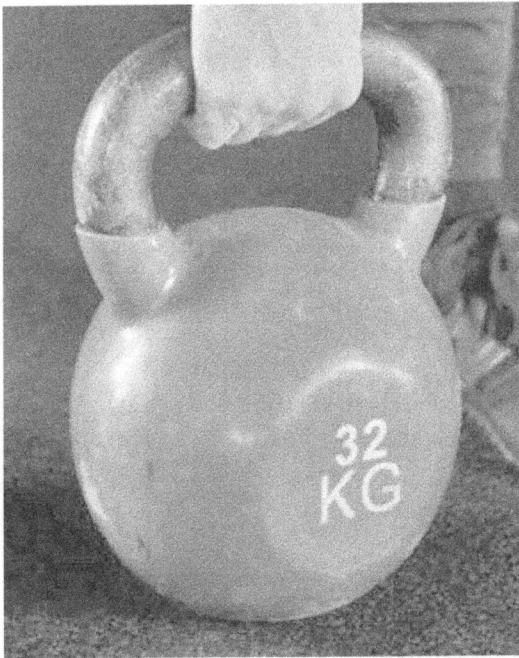

A kettlebell

The guideline for men

BMI

Your body is a combination of tissue, bone, water, muscle, and fat. Most of us have more fat than we need, and that can be very dangerous. Too much fat increases the risk of many illnesses, like heart disease, type 2 diabetes, high blood pressure, stroke, and even some forms of cancer.

According to the National Institutes of Health, losing as little as 5% of your body weight reduces your chances of developing a serious illness.

When you consume more calories than you burn, the extra calories are stored as fat. Genes are also a factor; some bodies simply make more fat than others. Gender matters, too. Men tend to pack extra fat around their gut; women usually carry it in their behinds until menopause causes an accumulation of fat around the middle.

How much fat is too much? To find out, you may want to find out your body mass index, or BMI. The BMI isn't foolproof; it sometimes miscalculates body fat in athletes, but it does present a safe guideline.

Body Mass Index (BMI) is a method of calculating body fat based on height and weight. It also measures your fitness level.

Sample guide bellow:

Underweight: BMI below 18.5
Normal: 18.5 to 24.9
Overweight: 25 to 29.9
Obese: 30 and above

Typically, you tend to lose fat first where you gained it last. While you can't reduce fat in just one area, you can replace flab with strong, sexy muscles through exercise and weight training.

The weight-standard

Overweight means a weight that is 10–20% greater than normal.

Obese people weigh 20% more than normal people.

Everybody, in reality, has a different layout for their calories burned, storage, and muscle building individuality. Maybe there is a mistake in these standards.

Don't Be a Slave to the Scale: Yes, weighing yourself every day will help keep you informed and on track. However, health and fitness are more than just a number.

Concentrate on exercising, eating a healthy diet, how you look in the mirror and how your clothes fit you.

Guidelines for women

HEIGHT	WEIGHT															
	100	110	120	130	140	150	160	170	180	190	200	210	220	230	240	250
5'0"	20	21	23	25	27	29	31	33	35	37	39	41	43	45	47	49
5'1"	19	21	23	25	26	28	30	32	34	36	38	40	42	43	45	47
5'2"	18	20	22	24	26	27	29	31	33	35	37	38	40	42	44	46
5'3"	18	19	21	23	25	27	28	30	32	34	35	37	39	41	43	44
5'4"	17	19	21	22	24	26	27	29	31	33	34	36	38	39	41	43
5'5"	17	18	20	22	23	25	27	28	30	32	33	35	37	38	40	42
5'6"	16	18	19	21	23	24	26	27	29	31	32	34	36	37	39	40
5'7"	16	17	19	20	22	23	25	27	28	30	31	33	34	36	38	39
5'8"	15	17	18	20	21	23	24	26	27	29	30	32	33	35	36	38
5'9"	15	16	18	19	21	22	24	25	27	28	30	31	32	34	35	37
5'10"	14	16	17	19	20	22	23	24	26	27	29	30	32	33	34	36
5'11"	14	15	17	18	20	21	22	24	25	26	27	28	30	32	33	35
6'0"	14	15	16	18	19	20	22	23	24	26	27	28	30	31	33	34
6'1"	13	15	16	17	18	20	21	22	24	25	26	28	29	30	32	33
6'2"	13	14	15	17	18	19	21	22	23	24	26	27	28	30	31	32
6'3"	12	14	15	16	17	19	20	21	22	24	25	26	27	29	30	31
6'4"	12	13	15	16	17	18	19	21	22	23	24	26	27	28	29	30

According to the CDC-Centers for Disease Control and Prevention, BMI is calculated the same way for both adults and children. The calculation is based on the following formulas: Because the calculation requires only height and weight, BMI is an inexpensive and easy tool.

Poundage and length

[weight (pounds)/height (inches)]$^{703 \times 2 =}$

By dividing weight in pounds (lbs) by height in inches (in) squared and multiplying by 703.

Example: Weight = 150 lbs., Height = 5'5" (65").

[150 (65) 2] multiplied by 703 equals 24.96.**Kilograms and meters (or centimeters) are both units of measurement.**

Second, [body mass index (BMI) / height (m)]

With the metric system, the formula for BMI is weight in kilograms divided by height in meters squared. Because height is commonly measured in centimeters, divide height in centimeters by 100 to obtain height in meters.

Example: weight = 68 kg, height = 165 cm (1.65 m).
Calculation: 68 (1.65) = 24.98

Other methods for measuring weight
In addition to BMI, women can use other methods to understand their weight and body composition. These include:

Waist circumference:
This method measures belly fat. People can calculate the circumference of their waist using a soft tape measure.

Waist-to-hip ratio (WHR)
This system also measures abdominal fat. Individuals can estimate their WHR by dividing their waist measurement by the circumference of their hips.
Diagnostic tests that a doctor may perform include

Densitometry: This consists of a doctor measuring someone's body weight while they are in water. This test, densitometry, generally takes place in a research setting.

- **Dual energy X-ray absorptiometry:** X-rays move through fat, muscle, and bone at different rates. This method facilitates two low-level X-rays through the body to calculate relative percentages.

- **Bioelectrical impedance (BIA):** BIA estimates someone's body fat by passing a low-level electric current through the body.

- **Isotope dilution:** A person in this test drinks water that contains isotopes and then provides samples of bodily fluids.

BMI is still a convenient and useful tool for measuring overall body weight.

Body Type-BMI

Bodybuilding champions, gyms, and hospitals measure body-fat percentages with skin-pinching calipers. You should do it too.

You don't need a scale.

To find your BMI, divide your weight in pounds by your height in inches, then multiply that by 703. A BMI of 25 to 29.99 is considered high-risk for women.

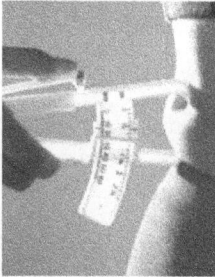

There are other tests to measure your BMI, like submerging your body underwater, but it is not necessary to do this expensive test. The one with the caliper is good enough.

This guide is not 100% correct, but it does provide guidelines.

Here are some guide numbers:

BMI
1-Underweight: below 18.5

2-Normal: 18.4 to 24.7

3-Overweight: 25 to 29.

4- Obese: 30 and higher

Three male Body Types

1-The Ectomorph

They have fast metabolisms, slim bodies, long arms, a little fat, are nervous and talkative, and eat whatever they want.

2-The Mesomorph

These are like natural-born athletes; wide shoulders, husky muscular bodies, kind of athletic, very strong, big chest, very long body.

Muscle size comes easily and progresses fast on any exercise.

We call them the fast gainers.

3-The Endomorph

These have a slow metabolism, a short neck, wide hips, and a tendency to store lots of fat in a pear-shaped body.

Goals

1-Add some body weight. They must keep working the big muscles.

2- This body type won't have any problems adding muscles. This body type is kind of bulky, and should pay attention to its shape.

This type will grow fast.

3-This body type has high fat storage, so they need to do a lot of cardio. It is important to pay attention to what they eat and the quantity.

ILLUSTRATION

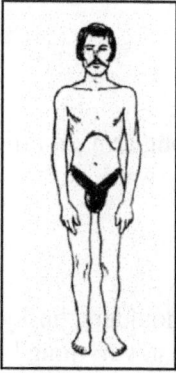

THE ECTOMORPH

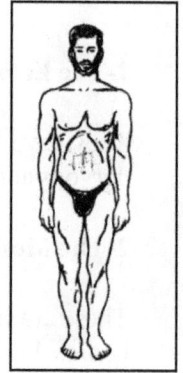

THE MESOMORPH

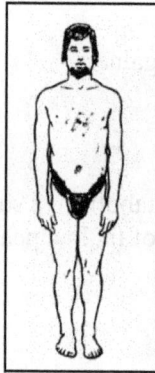

THE ENDOMORPH

You are probably a combination of one or two, sometimes even three, types. There are many different ways to find out what type you are. For example, there are height and weight tables. These tables, however, only measure weight and don't look into body composition.

Secondly, you can have someone use the skin fold measurement test. This is a simple way to assess body fat using skin-fold calipers that test skin and fat at various sites on your body. There's also underwater weighing, which is the most accurate way to evaluate fat to muscle ratio. However, it's kind of expensive. Finally, you can use the most common one, which is to look in the mirror.

Fat-burning furnace

Here are the six worst things you can do if you want to ignite your body's own fat-burning furnace and get lean, strong, and totally ripped in less time:

Mistake # 1

Doing Isolated Exercises

Doing isolated movements like bicep curls and triceps kick-backs will not get you any significant results. One-muscle-at-a-time simply doesn't stimulate sufficient muscle fibers to build lean muscle or maximize your calorie burn.

Mistake # 2

Working Out With Machines

Mistake # 3

Long Sessions of Cardio

You need to do cardio if you want to lose weight and burn fat, but be careful about pounding the pavement with sore feet.

Mistake # 4

Doing Crunches & Sit-Ups to Get 6-Pack Ab

Doing traditional ab exercises like crunches and sit-ups will not get you a six pack. They don't make your abs get any more defined and they definitely don't burn any fat.

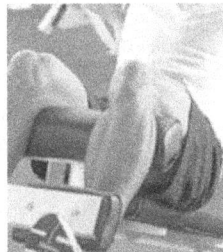

Mistake# 5

Repeating the Same Workouts Over and Over

Stop doing the same old workouts that haven't gotten you any results. Repeating the same workouts over and over is a surefire way to never get results. If you want to keep making improvements and keep seeing changes in your body, you've got to start switching things up.

Mistake# 6

Doing long workouts

Longer workouts do not give you faster results. The trick is shorter, faster, and more intensive workouts. Be wary of doing too much aerobics because it will interfere with muscle development. Your knees might begin to show the strain, and your feet, ankles, or hips might begin to show the pounding.

Make sure to wear good sneakers. We lose muscle regularly each year after our mid-20s, and running is not a muscle builder after the initial conditioning period.

Swimming program

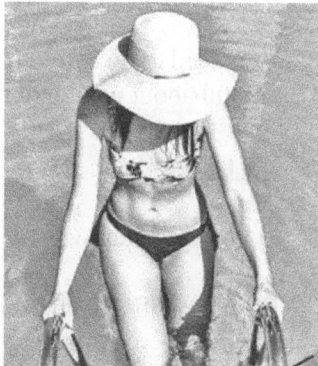

Experts claim that the body retains layers of fat under the skin to protect it from the water temperature. I really believe, like many experts, that swimming is an opposing muscle-building activity. Swimming naturally encourages the body to be strong and buoyant, increasing internal fat and surface fat. Adding the swimmer's buoyancy factor might be a hard problem to overcome, and achieve the desirable six-pack.

In other words, I believe like experts do that swimming make you fat. Give it a try and see if it works for you.

Don't Recline After You Dine

If you lie down right after eating, it can make it more challenging for your body to digest the food you just ate. This can lead to an increase in intestinal bloating and gas production. Instead, sit upright or stand for at least an hour after eating a meal before you lie down.

Walk Off Your Meal

A brief walk after eating can speed intestinal transit, increase the rate of digestion, and cut down on gas production.

No to Sodas

Sodas and carbonated drinks are already infused with gas. You're introducing gas into your digestive tract. To avoid gas problems, avoid carbonated beverages. Also avoid many fruit juices.

Avoid cold drinks.

Drinking cold drinks with a meal can slow down your body's digestive actions. In addition, the cold temperature of the drinks may cause digestive discomfort and gas. Skip the ice and sip a room-temperature beverage. Forget about using a straw, says Lynne Crosby, author of Belly Fat for Dummies and a spokeswoman for the Academy of Nutrition and Dietetics. Instead, switch to sipping from a glass to cut down on the amount of air you swallow.

Preventing Gas

Stay away from foods as well as gum or candy with sorbitol as a sweetener. This sugar sweetener is often poorly digested. Mannitol, another sugar usually found in sugar-free mints and gum. Avoid talking too much while eating to reduce the amount of air you swallow.

> *"If you wish to live long, take a walk after meal."*
> *Húo dào jǐu shí jǐu*

Crash Diets

Crash diets and diets don't work. If you restrict calories, a diet low in calories will cause muscle loss and put a stop to your fat-burning metabolism, causing you to gain all the weight back after you get back to your normal eating. Yoyo theory, remember?

To develop a bikini body, you don't need to work at 100% intensity. If you're aiming for a perfect bikini body, lean and tight with curves in all the right places, this plan is for you.

Exercising While Dieting

1-Order a salad with no dressing.

2-Order a grilled chicken breast, fish, or a lean cut of beef.

3-Have a cheat meal once in a while at your favorite restaurant.

Yogurt: These cultures, or active bacteria, aid in digestion, keeping your inner workings effective. Yogurt is a dairy product that will help fight lactose intolerance because of the natural presence of lactase, an enzyme that assists in digesting lactose.

Broccoli delivers vitamin C, calcium, and zinc.

Spinach helps fight ovarian cancer, and the ability to carry oxygen from the lungs to the muscles.

Bananas will balance potassium and electrolytes. help muscle contractions during exercise.

Fatty Fish: Findings have revealed that fish oil helps fight joint stiffness and muscle fatigue.

Turkey contains selenium and vitamin B6, which is good protein.

Drink a lot of water! This is especially important in the hot summer months. It keeps you hydrated and keeps your system flushed.

WATER

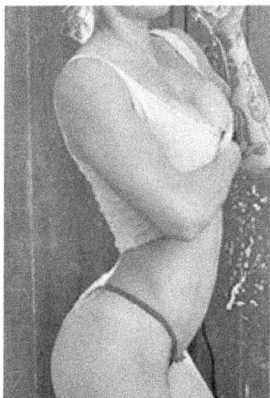

Drink a glass of water before every meal. In several findings of weight loss in overweight adults, those who drank water before eating a meal regularly ingested fewer calories and saw improved weight loss results.

Cold water speeds up your metabolism. In research on water-induced thermogenesis, scientists learned that drinking water triggered an increase in energy expenditure in both men and women, likely caused by the efforts to warm the water to body temperature.

The effects of elevated metabolism started about 10 minutes after drinking the water and peaked at 30-40 minutes after drinking. Drink water and cut your salt intake to lose water weight. Reducing the quantity of dietary salt you ingest can help you lose water weight quickly, particularly when combined with an increase in daily water intake.

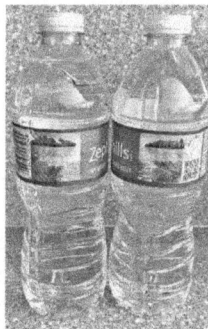

Water is a very essential nutrient. Two thirds of the human body is water. Men and women can only live a few days without water.

The amount of water the body loses from perspiration, respiration and elimination is about 2-3 quarts a day. Water helps cool the body down and provides the body with minerals.

Not having enough water can and will cause many problems. Drink enough water so your urine is clear. Water makes up about 80 percent of the muscles and about 60 percent of the body.

How much water you need depends on your size. A 180-pound person needs about four quarts or more per day. More than two quarts of water should be consumed. Drink plenty of water every day, eight glasses or more. Water clears, dissolves, and eliminates toxins, relieves constipation, and absorbs nutrients. The role of water in maintaining good health has been recognized since ancient times. Water keeps the skin healthy, the organs fed with blood and nutrients, and the brain functioning.

Hippo Crates, the Father of Medicine, recommended an increase in water consumption. Also, there is now evidence that cold water makes you lose weight. So drink a lot of water, before working out, during, and after you are done exercising. It's necessary for all your organs. Don't neglect it.

Keep in mind that enhanced waters with vitamins, etc., are loaded most of the time with sugar. Drink more than you need. Dehydration is serious.

Some Symptoms of dehydration are:

Dry mouth	Fatigue
Headache	Dim vision
Dizziness	Clumsiness

When you have just completed your morning workout, the first thing you should do is drink a glass of water, whether you are thirsty or not, before you take your training clothes off. I personally don't drink this water cold; I drink it like an animal does, just like ambient water.

Clues that you need water are: sweaty clothes, high humidity, even fatigue. Water is the most important nutrient your body needs to stay healthy, especially in the heat of the summer. Water regulates the body's temperature and transports nutrients. The problem is that most people don't drink enough. Drinking eight 8-ounce glasses of water daily is the minimum standard recommendation; drink more if you exercise. It is a good idea to drink one glass when you wake up in the morning and another just before you go to bed.

Drink plenty of water throughout the day

Food Substitutions

Make Smart Food Substitutions: Make it simple to cut calories while still enjoying your favorite foods: Use skim milk instead of 2%, order grilled chicken instead of crispy, and eat yogurt instead of ice cream.

This approach can be adjusted to any cuisine.

Portion size counts with supersized French fries. According to the National Institutes of Health, 20 years ago, a typical muffin weighed 1.5 ounces and had 210 calories.

Today it's 4 ounces and 500 calories. Two slices of pepperoni pizza used to be 500 calories. Now they're 850. At least 100 calories are saved by eating a 3-ounce bagel instead of a 4-ounce one.

Beware of Condiments: Those little sauces and creams seem so harmless, but look out. Use low-fat whipped cream cheese on your bagel instead of full-fat, non-whipped cream cheese.

Watch Out for Toppings, Dressings, and Dips. Salads look so healthy, but they can be packed with hidden calories.

Use a low-fat dressing or switch to a vinaigrette. And ditch the croutons!

Drink responsibly; alcohol can be another source of hidden calories. For health reasons as well as a way to cut calories, women should have no more than one drink a day, while men should stop at two. Reduce your alcohol consumption by one drink and you've saved yourself 100 calories.

Replace pasta with whole grain pasta or vegetables, such as spaghetti.

If you want to lose weight and keep it off without making sacrifices, you need to eat the right foods. What are the right foods?

Simple, whole foods. Try eating foods as close to their natural state as you can.

If you can eat organic foods, food that is certified organic must meet strict criteria and follow rules like how it is grown, packaged, stored, and shipped.

Remember, different countries may have different standards.

In the case of poultry, hormones may be used to grow the chickens. Not everything you eat has to be organic.

If you want to lose weight, you have to burn more calories in a day than you consume. That's the reality.

If your goal is to lose weight, stop eating when you feel about 75% full. You don't have to feel stuffed. Eat slowly and have a glass of water.

4 times per day

You should eat four times per day: breakfast, lunch, snack, and dinner. Your biggest meals should be breakfast and an early dinner, plus a small snack during the day. Your last meal should be at least two hours before you go to bed.

You must find the right time for dinner, because it is hard to sleep when you are hungry. The secret to losing weight is portion control, eating whole foods, and leaving some food on the plate without stuffing yourself.

Best choices:
Lean meat
Fish
Lean poultry
Peas, beans
Raw nuts

Avoid the trap.

Quick service restaurants

Fried fish and meat

Processed meats like bacon and hot dogs.

Chips, cakes, doughnuts, crackers

Eat all the colors of vegetables; green, yellow, red, orange, and purple. Try to eat them fresh, but you can eat them frozen too. Some diets call for limiting carbohydrates, but you need carbohydrates in your diet for your body to function properly.

You need protein, carbohydrates, and fat. I know you are thinking fat. No, fat won't make you fat; cutting fat won't disrupt your weight loss plan.

There are three types of fats: unsaturated fats (good), saturated fats (kind of bad) and trans fats (really bad). These bad fats can clog your arteries, give your heart disease, and raise your cholesterol level (LDL).

Sugar

It is bad for your waistline. You should avoid refined sugar as much as possible, but it is impossible to completely avoid it. Go easy on unnatural sugar, but you can have it in fruits and vegetables. If you really need to lose weight, I would cut refined, processed sugar from your diet.

"All disease starts in the guts"
Hippocrates

Amino Acids

They are components of protein. Some are produced by the body, others must be taken from food. There are 22 amino acids.

Alanine Aid the immune system. Regulate the metabolism.

Arginine tones muscles, helps sperm in males, and increases physical and mental alertness.

Sodium Aspartate Excellent for the immune system.

Carnitine Use it for intense workouts, reduce angina attacks, and help liver and kidney illness.

Cysteine/Cystine Antioxidants-anti-aging.

Gamma-aminobutyric acid Assist nerves in reaching the brain.

Glutamic acid and glutamine improve brain functions.

Glutathione is an anti-tumor agent- good for the respiratory system.

Glycine stimulates the brain, helping with a swollen prostate.

Histidine helps arthritis by dilatation of blood vessels.

Ornithine is a muscle-building substance.

Prolone helps with thinking ability.

Serine generates cellular energy and helps with pain

Taurine supports the heart and central nervous system.

Tyrosine Adjust your emotional behavior.

Valine is essential for positive hydrogen balance in the body.

Vitamins

There are two kinds of vitamins: water-soluble and fat-soluble. Water- solvable are flushed out in the urine. The other kind of vitamin, fat-soluble, is stored in the body. There are 23 classified vitamins; they are organic and found in living things. Each one performs different functions in the human body. Make sure you eat or take them. Vitamins are required by the human body.

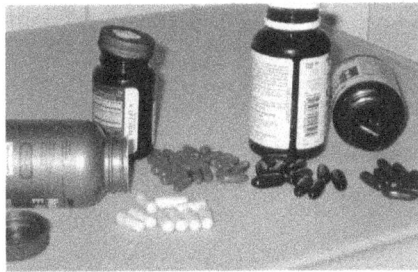

Carbohydrates

Carbohydrates develop into glycogen. Glycogen is fuel or energy used by the body to move muscles into action. It's the main source of fuel for your muscles. It's excellent for the recuperation process. Your body is in need of it after working out. It's a big part of the American diet. Very important to bodybuilders' training.

Proteins

The most important source for a bodybuilder is called the "king's blocks of life." They add weight, muscle, and bulk, which are very essential for growth. Words derived from the Greek language The American College of Sports Medicine advises between 1.4 and 2 grams of protein per kilo of bodyweight each day. I really don't believe too much in using extra protein powder. I have used it sparingly, but never for too long.

Extra protein is a waste of money, and it might be hard on your kidneys. There are two kinds: vegetable and animal. The late Mike Mentzer agreed with me on this one. The amount of protein a man or a bodybuilder requires depends on his size, work, and the kind of training he does.

135

Fats

The body's reserve energy supply. Some come from animal sources. This is bad fat. Fatty acids are insoluble in water. Fats carry the fat-soluble vitamin. Olive oil, corn oil, etc. are much better.

Protein + Strength Training

A high-protein regimen combined with strength training will help people gain muscle mass and lose body weight.

Experts claim that the combination is about four grams of carbs for every gram of protein.

Aerobics, kickboxing, and fat

For activities that involve repetitive joint action, monounsaturated fats from fish, nuts, seeds, canola, olive, and peanut oils can help lubricate the joints while also providing high-quality protein to power you through a workout.

Bill Wallace, a karate champion, claimed that consuming oil lubricated his joints and kept them in top notch for kicking.

An added benefit is that these fats help to reduce post-workout soreness and stiffness. I read and learned this many years ago from karate champion Bill Wallace.

Vitamins won't function without minerals

Vitamins:

Vitamin A-Beta Carotene A fat-soluble vitamin It is good for your vision, skin, and mucous membranes.
1,000 milligrams daily.

The B-Complex It's good for the immune system, nervous system, and heart. It is also an anti-stress and mood enhancer.

B-I-Thiamine Normal digestion and formation of blood
200-300 mg daily.

Riboflavin B-2 carries the energy required for the life of cells.
200-300.

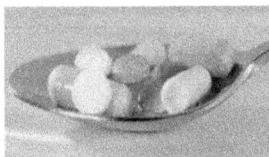

B-3 Niacin necessary for energy, to reduce bad cholesterol (LDL) and raise good cholesterol (HDL).
50-100 mg daily

Pantothenic acid (B-5) is required to produce energy and fight microbes and stress. It's also known as the anti-stress vitamin.
300-1,000 mg. daily

Pyridoxine B-6 necessary for the metabolism of amino acids. It fights fatigue, anemia, kidney stones, and some neurological symptoms.
50 mg. daily.

Folic acid helps the production of red blood cells to carry oxygen to the cells, important for maintaining nucleic acids.
400 mg per day.

Cyanocobalamin B-12 is essential for the formation of red blood cells, normal growth, and the nervous system.
100–200 mg daily.

B-15-Pangamic Acid an antioxidant- helps recover from fatigue 500–1,000 mg per day

Inositol it's good for hair, neurological disease, lowering cholesterol levels, protecting the heart.
300-400 mg per day

Biotin Build protein, white blood cells, fight germs, and aid immune systems.300 mg daily.

Paba Formation of blood cells, it's good for sunscreen, reversing gray hair- 30 mg daily.

Vitamin C-Ascorbic Acid Slows arteriosclerosis, blood clots, shortens duration of colds, in others words, it boosts immunity.
60 milligrams daily

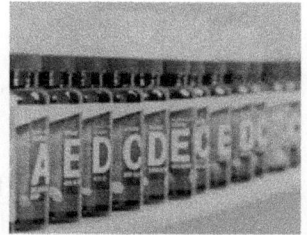

Vitamin D-Calciferol for strong bones, teeth, and the healthy heart.
400-1,000 IU per day

Vitamin E-Tocopherol Reduces risk of heart disease, cancer, and Alzheimer's. An antioxidant that slows the aging process, helps with degenerative diseases, and infections, excellent.
400 internationally distributed units

Vitamin K aids in blood clotting and liver function.
50-100 mcg per day

Vitamin P-Bioflavonoids- It's good for hypertension, infections, colds, and gum infections 10-20 mg daily.

Vitamin K Aids in blood clotting, important in liver function.
50-100 mcg daily

Vitamin P-Bioflavonoids-Rutin Good for the circulation- prevents blood clots 10-20 mg daily.

Minerals

Minerals are a combination of protein, fats, and carbohydrates. They are essential in a person's diet, especially for a bodybuilder. Vitamins won't function without minerals. Minerals work together with hormones, enzymes, amino acids, and vitamins. The body must use minerals to maintain itself. As a result, it is critical to include minerals in your diet.

Boron

It helps with bone loss in women.

Chromium

It will lower cholesterol, give you energy, help you gain muscle and lose fat.

Calcium

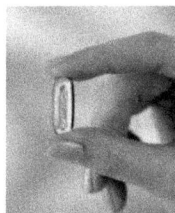

It strengthens bones and teeth and aids in blood clotting. It also regulates the heart and is good for vitality and energy.

Cobalt

Needed to produce red blood cells to stimulate growth.

Fluoride

It protects your teeth.

Iodine

Healthy hair, nails, and teeth are necessary for the thyroid gland, growth, and energy.

Iron

Helps to make hemoglobin, which carries oxygen into the blood and can be harmful.

Magnesium

It regulates heartbeats and helps regulate high blood pressure.

Manganese

Preserves sex hormone, nerves, and brain

Potassium

It balances water in the body, helps with high blood pressure and energy levels.

Selenium

It helps the immune system, body growth, and aging.

Sodium

It balances water in the muscles and body. It's known as salt.

Sulfur

It helps the liver and gives you shiny hair, which is important for nice skin.

Vanadium

It helps muscles develop and grow, and also helps teeth and bones.

Zinc

Aids in tissue functions, impotence, diseases, and fertility. Zinc is necessary for the function of the prostate gland.

Fiber

There are two kinds of fiber: soluble and insoluble. Soluble is found in fruits, insoluble in wheat and cereals. Both are low in fat, help with regularity, and are good for cholesterol and high blood pressure. It will lower your risk of colon cancer.

Enzymes

A complex protein is necessary for the digestion process. Some of the best are bromelain and papain.

The sun's vitamin D?

As needed by the human body, you need to be exposed for 15–30 minutes a day to activate enzymes, stimulate hormone production, and improve nutrient absorption. But the sun is also responsible for wrinkling. Skin will become old-looking. Keep it in mind and stay in the shade to look young.

Consider this: maximize your muscular gains.

Warming Up

The first and most important rule is to avoid strain and injury. Spend some time on your preferred cardio to elevate your heart rate and warm the muscles. Always begin with lighter weights to make sure your muscles get used to the movement before using heavier weights.

Don't Overdo It.

Most people, including you, are probably familiar with the expression, "No pain, no gain." You must be careful; working a muscle to exhaustion can be counter-productive because it increases recovery time and you take the chance of getting an injury.

Another common mistake made by beginners to the gym is lifting too much weight too fast without giving the body time to get used to the work load.

Supplements

We live in a culture of quick fixes, and people want to bulk up or lose weight now, in this moment, tomorrow. There are many supplements that promise you almost instant results. This is not true. There are many incredible, good products out there, but they need time to work.

Don't be fooled into thinking that simply taking some pills will make you muscular. Your body needs constant nourishment to ensure an effective workout. Just make sure to get enough protein, fat, and carbohydrates.

Sleeping

Sleep is essential for growing muscles, which actually recover during sleep. The average person needs seven to nine hours of sleep every 24 hours.

Laying down

Lying down after eating is not a good idea. It will become difficult to digest the food you just ate, and you will experience increased intestinal bloating and gas production. It is better to stand, sit upright after eating, or take a 3-minute walk before you lie down.

A brief walk after eating is proven to increase digestion, reduce gas production, and also, by doing this, burn off some of the calories you just ate.

Sodas are not permitted.

Sodas and carbonated beverages that are gaseous will cause gas in your digestive area. Stop these drinks to avoid an irritating gas condition.You can also prevent gas by limiting your talking while you are having lunch or dinner, so you cut down on the amount of air you ingest when you eat.

Stay away from cold drinks.

Cold drinks most likely give you digestive discomfort and gas. People who drink cold beverages with meals probably slow down their body's digestive actions and eliminate cold drinks.

Belly Fat for Dummies author and a spokeswoman for the Academy of Nutrition and Dietetics. I said, "Forget about using a straw; instead, switch to sipping from a glass to cut down on the amount of air you swallow."

Imitated Sweeteners

Stay away from gum or candy with sorbitol as a sweetener. This sweetener is often badly assimilated. Mannitol is another that is frequently found in sugar-free mints and gum, and will cause excessive gas in some people.

143

Fitness- Partner-Advantages

When you exercise with a partner, you are more likely to stick to your workout routine and perform better and archive better results than those who go it alone.

Here are four fitness buddy advantages:

Responsibility:
When someone waits for you at the gym or at the park, it is easier to stay in track.

Support:
A good partner will keep you interested.

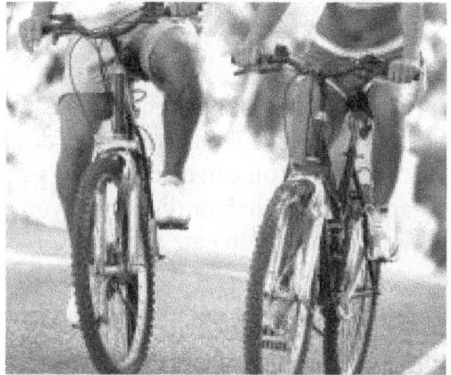

Buddy Competition: Contest among friends are a good way to keep going.

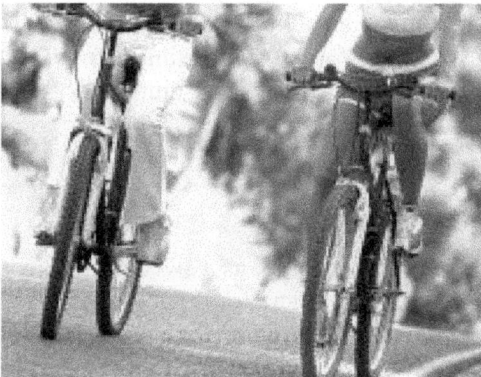

Social Clubs:
Groups are a perfect way to take walks together and motivate one another.

Strands/Cable/spring chest expander routine

The chest expander equipment was invented in the late 1800's. The design consists of two handles attached by coils of springs that create resistance. The conventional version is the metal spring version, and today's chest expanders are made with adjustable rubber cables instead of metal springs. The rubber version can do the job of traditional spring-based chest expanders.

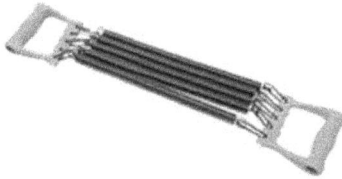

Cable/spring workouts are great when you are on vacation. They are compact, portable, and they don't take much space. They do not weigh anything, can be carried in a small handbag, and do not make any noise. You can do it in a resort, park, or stairs; they work your muscles in a different way, with a greater range of motion than traditional weights. The most imperative thing about working out with cables is to be regular. You also must be intelligent. Don't overdo it at the beginning.

I received my first set of springs back when I was only 12 years old, and throughout my life I have used them from time to time. I still own two complete sets of spring chest expanders. After more than 60 years, I am a real fan of these old-school tools, like expanders and power twisters.

The chest expander is used to target the chest muscles. It can also be used to exercise the arms and back as well. When you work out, find the right time when you don't get any interruptions. Avoid exercising after a meal, particularly after a heavy one. Use as many cables/springs as you can, but make sure you can do the recommended repetitions.

Use the correct form. Your exercises must be done correctly. You will build muscles and tone if you work out every day.

For good symmetry, exercise both sides of your body similarly. Concentrate on the muscles you are working out. Exercise without straining.

The chest expander can be used to increase the size of your chest muscles.

The National Academy of Sports Medicine (NASM) recommends doing 8 to 12reps.

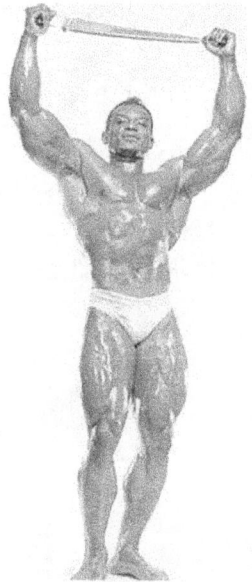

1-Cable Chest Pull

Champion Sergio Oliva

Chest -Shoulders

Hold the spring at arm's length in front of your body, draw each hand until it's directly under your shoulders while taking a deep breath. Repeat for 8 reps

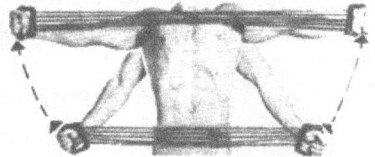

2-Curl

Biceps

Holding cables to the side of your body, with arm straight. Bend the arm at the elbow, slowly bringing the hand to the shoulder. Return slowly to beginning position and repeat for 8 reps.

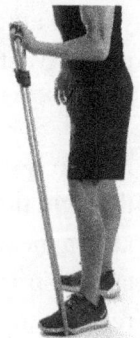

3- Press & Raise Overhead

Shoulder-Chest

Hold the cable/spring directly in front of you. Slowly raise it out and upward to complete extension, raising the cables above your head. Return slowly and repeat for a total of 8 reps.

4-Diagonal Chest

One hand holds the cable straight above the head and the other is fully bent at the chest with the back of the hand.

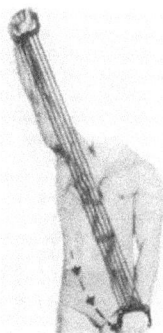

Slowly press the arm straight to the side, keeping the upright straight arm straight.

Repeat for 8 reps.

Chest

5- Triceps push down

Holding the springs vertical in front of you, push down with the other hand to hit the triceps.

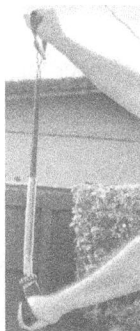

Return slowly and repeat for 8 reps.

6-Cable behind Neck-Press Out

Shoulder and back

With your arms fully bend and spring/cables behind your neck, slowly press your arms out to shoulder level, and slowly return.

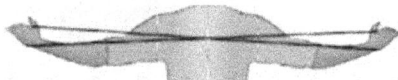

Repeat for 8 reps.

7-**Bench Press**-with band around your upper body, press out and extend both arms, relax and repeat .Chest, shoulders, arms- and repeat for 8 reps.

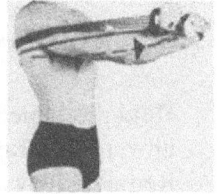

Use as many cable/springs as will allow doing 8 reps. Adjust the cables of the chest expander as needed. As you progress you can add reps, and later on, ad cables or springs.

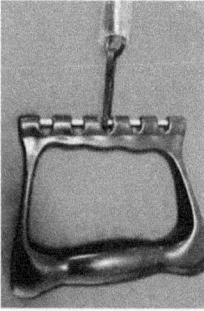

I guarantee you, by the time you are using 4 or 5 cables or springs for 15 reps on each exercise, you will not only look stronger, but you will be also stronger, toned, symmetrical and more muscular.

Be very careful. Make sure the springs or cables are attached correctly before beginning your workout. An unexpected mistake can cause you to lose a spring or rubber and hit your head, face or eye, or you can lose grip on one of the handles, which can result in injury. I advise you to always wear protective glasses for safety. Be careful with the springs that press against your skin.

Rubber bands can do the job of spring-based chest expanders, but steel spring expanders are a better choice.

Cable/springs workouts are excellent for when traveling and it's impossible to visit the gym, or you are limited in space to keep any kind of equipment.

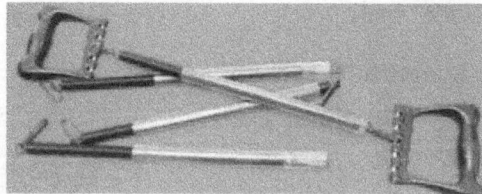

SPRING CHEST ESPANDER

148

Isometric-Charles Atlas Exercises

Isometric exercises are anaerobic and involve the contraction of muscles without any movement in the surrounding joints. This is a type of static strength training that activates or contracts muscles without visible movement of the body.

For years, doctors believed that these kinds of exercises increased blood pressure. Talk to your doctor before you start doing isometrics, just in case.

When doing isometric exercises, the natural tendency is to hold your breath. Don't, and exhale before you tense up your muscles.

According to the Mayo Clinic, isometric exercises are often prescribed as a path to healing for arthritis and rotor cuff injuries.

Neck exercise: Place both palms on your brow. Push your head forward while you push your palms back to resist the movement. Hold for 10 seconds.

Place your hand behind your head, push your head back, and repeat. Hold for 10 seconds.

Chest-Press hands with elbows out against each other, hold for a few seconds, relax, and repeat.

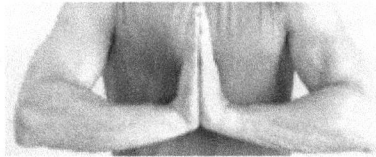

Chest-Press hand low in front of chest with elbows out, hold for a few seconds, repeat.

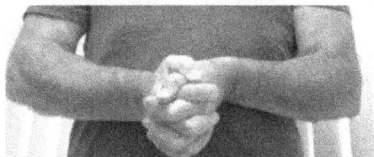

Shoulders-Stand inside a door frame, press your back hands against the frame for a few seconds, repeat.

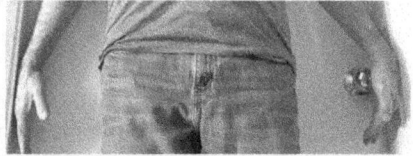

Shoulders- Stand against a wall. Press your elbows back against the wall, hold for a few seconds and repeat.

Arms-Biceps-Curl
Bend arm at the elbows, hold hand with the other hand, press down while resisting with the other hand.

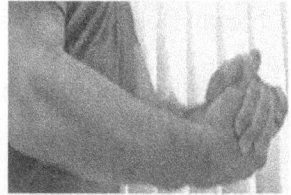

Arms Triceps- Press Down
Bend the arm at the elbow, with hand facing down. Place hand over the other hand, press down while you resisting with the other hand. Repeat.

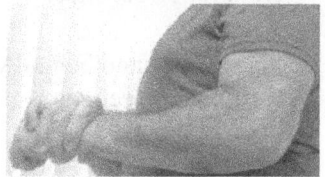

Back/Lats
Seat, as you pull your leg out, you resist with both of your arms, concentrating on your lats. Repeat with other leg.

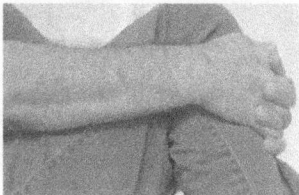
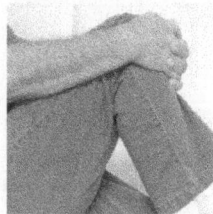

Start   Finished

Legs Curls-Hamstring

Stand up and bend your legs backward. Hold your feet and pull your leg up with your hand as you resist with your leg. Repeat.

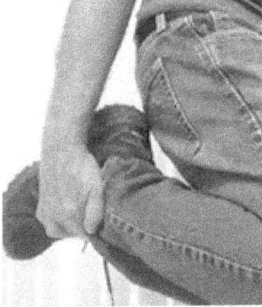

Start

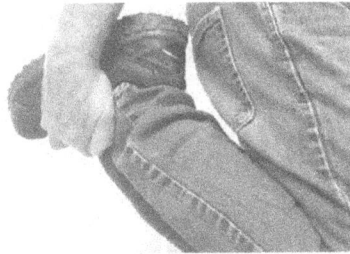

Finish

Calf /Standing

Standing on a piece of wood, step, or block, lower your feet down on the step, stretching both heels, and then raising them as high as you can. Repeat up and down.

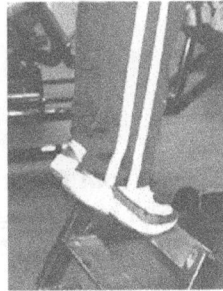

Power Twister

The Power Twist is extremely effective. The only drawback is adjusting the resistance. But you can adjust the resistance by just moving your grip, close or wide, or also by moving the Power Twist away or close to your body.

Get the best pump you've ever felt! You can develop your chest, back, shoulders, and arms into rippling muscle builder. It's the perfect device to use at the office or take along when you travel. There is nothing to remove, add or put together.

Chest, Shoulders, Traps, Arms

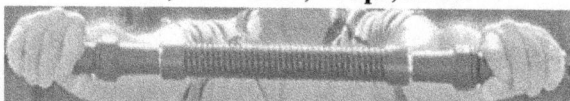

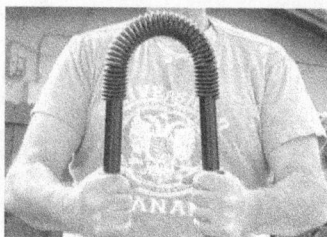

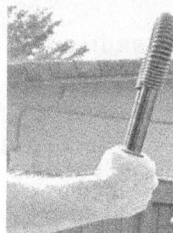

1-Front Chest
Star by holding the Power Twist in front of chest, gripping and holding the handles at 90% bend in your elbows. Bend the Twist while focusing and squeezing the chest muscle.
Relax and repeat.

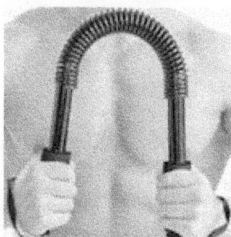

2- Burn-Front Chest
Star by holding the Power Twist in front of chest, gripping and holding the handles at 90% bend in elbows. Bend the Twist and do short reps, never going to the starting point, while focusing and squeezing the chest muscle. Relax and repeat.

3- Behind neck
Place the twist behind your neck, resting part of the twist on top of your shoulder by the neck. Bend the twist, relax, and repeat.

4- Arms
Star by holding the Power Twist in front of your chest, using an inside grip, bending the twist while focusing and squeezing the chest muscle, To make it harder, keep the twist away from your body. Relax and repeat.

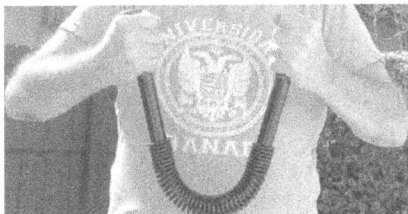

5- Bicep
Hold the twist upright, with one hand holding the top grip, while the other hand holds the bottom grip, and bend the twist from the top handle, like trying to touch one handle with the other. Concentrate and squeeze the biceps. Relax and repeat.

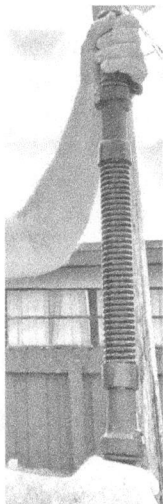

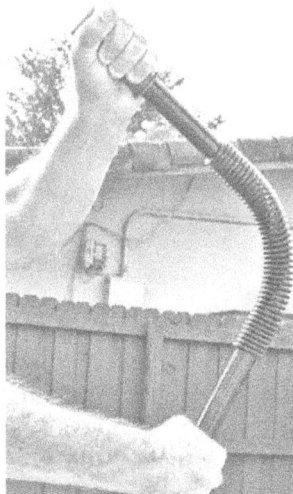

The greatest muscle builder you'll ever own
There is no reason to not train everywhere

Fit Bands

It is easy to start building muscles, with no attachments, no bolts, and no screws to assemble. Designed to be used in a few feet of space, it requires no maintenance and works quietly. It weighs ounces, so it builds a more muscular body quickly and economically in your own home. Bands can be use practically anywhere and at any time. Easy to take on a trip; no bulky equipment.

Always check your bands before use. If you detect any damage, do not use the band. Under no circumstances should you wrap your band around a sharp object. Drawbacks: A sudden snap of the band/spring can cause painful slaps and pinches, even face injuries. I advise you to always wear protective glasses for safety.

Pullup assist bands with differing resistance levels are the ideal exercise for building upper body strength and even lower body muscles. Pullup assist bands will help increase the number of unassisted pulls ups, it is also extremely versatile and can be used in other ways, including stretching, powerlifting, and mobility training.

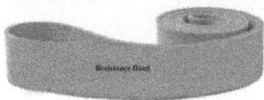

They're useful for warmups to stretch and strengthen your hamstrings, arms, and shoulders.

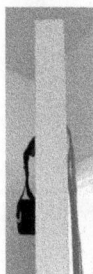

The door anchor is an essential tool for your home workouts. Slip between the hinges side of a door and securely close the door, and you are ready to go. You can place it on the top, halfway or at the bottom to hit the muscle from different angles.

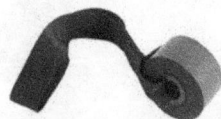

Always double check to make sure the door and anchor is safely in place before beginning any exercise. For safety reasons, you must use it against the way the door opens.

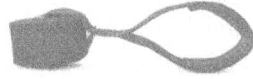

The Assist Band is ideal for:

Stretching, Powerlifting, Resistance Training.
Resistance Bands
Increased Power
Rehabilitates Injuries
When exercising the leg muscles
Great for assisted/pull-ups/chin-ups.
So you can do a variety of exercises.

Chest Pull: With band in front of you, arms extended, pull the band up using both hands at the same time you inhale deeply, return arms to the front as you exhale.
Chest, shoulders, arms-2sets of x 8 reps

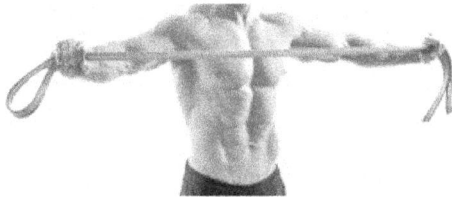

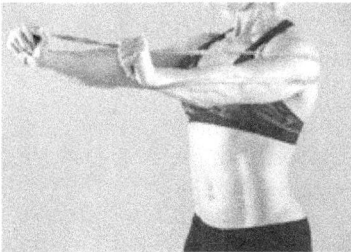

Bench Press: while wearing a band around your upper body, press out and extend both arms, relax and repeat. Chest, shoulders, arms. 2sets of x 8 reps

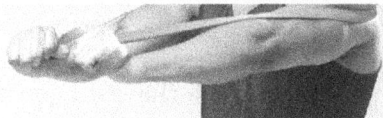

Push-ups: with the band across your upper back, extend your legs back in a straight line, lower yourself until your chest is inches from the floor, and then return to the starting position. Chest, arms.2 sets of x 8 reps.

Front Raises: Place one end of the band under each of your feet. Raise your arms directly up and forward, until they are parallel with the floor. Hold the top position for a second before gradually returning to the start position-Shoulder-2sets of x 8 reps

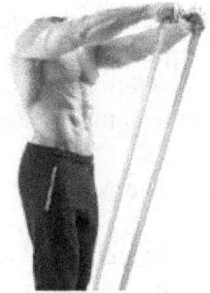

Upright Row: Hold the band in front of you by the waist in an underhand grip. Pull the band up to your chest, bringing your elbows high and out to the sides. Return to the starting position slowly.Shoulders-2 sets of x 8 reps

Exercises Lat Pull-down: Place the looped end of the band on a door anchor to hold the end of the band. You could Sit on the floor below the bar or door, or stand up if you use the top position. With the band in each hand securely closed, extend your arms over your head. From a fully extended position, pull the bands down toward your chest, moving your arms as far back as you can. Hold for a second and then slowly return to the start position. Back-2sets of x 8 reps.

Curls: Stand with feet shoulder width and hold the band in an underhand grip at waist level. Place the band under both feet and curl the band, bending your elbows up to your chest. Don't move your elbows from the sides and contract your biceps. Return slowly to the start position   Biceps-2sets of x 8 reps

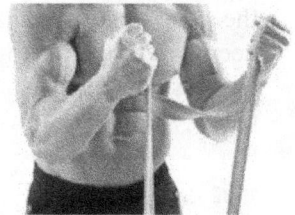

Lunges-Curls: As you do a lunge, do a curl at the same time, alternating with your left and right leg. Legs, arms, cardio.2sets x 8 reps

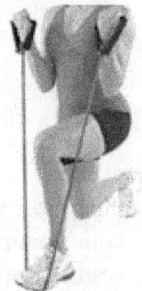

Triceps Push Downs: Loop the band over a high bar, a tree, or you can anchor the band in a doorway. Stand in front of the door with the band at chest level. Elbows clenched at your sides. Straighten your arms down by pushing to a fully extended position. Slowly raise your arms back up to the start position. Arms and legs- 2 x 8 rep sets

Press Down: With your hand holding the band on top of your shoulders, with your finger facing up, pull down and extend the band down to your upper chest. 2 sets of 8 reps

Squats: Place your feet slightly wider than shoulder width apart, with your toes pointing a little outwards. Place the band under both feet with the band around your neck, placing it on your trapezius, coming down in front of your shoulders.

Keep your butt back as you lower your body, lower down to a parallel squat position. Stand up slowly and repeat. 2 sets of 8 reps.

Deadlifting: Perform a deadlift by bending down to grab the band with an overhand grip, placing the band through your heels on both feet, pushing and rising to a standing position.

Hold the top position for a second and then slowly return to the starting position. For the entire body, do 2 sets of 8 reps.

Assist pull-ups: Secure the band to an overhead bar, place your feet, or if you prefer, your knees into the band, and pull yourself up doing a pull-up, assisted with the band.

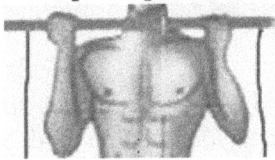

A perfect way to improve your Pull-ups range or get use to do them.

There are other types of bands, such as tubes, and here is a sample of them.

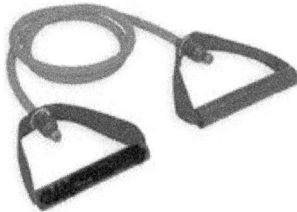

RESISTANCE BAND TENSION GUIDE

#1(orange) 0.51inch 15LB-35LB

#2(green) 0.87inch 25LB-65LB

#3(yellow) 1.12 inch 35LB-85LB

#4(red) 1.73 inch 50LB-125LB

ROTATOR CUFF EXERCISE

This is a simple exercise that is very important to prevent injuries. Every therapy center you visit includes this exercise as therapy. Arm rotation is an excellent exercise for the rotor cuff muscles and tendons and to stabilize the shoulder.

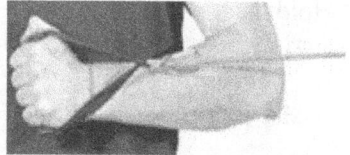

Attach the free end of the tube-band to a fixed support or rail, stand sideways to the rail, elbows bent, and rotate your hand inward, achieving the pronate action. Now redirect the band resistance and rotate your hands away from the body, to complete the supinate action.

Perform three sets of 25 reps on each hand, both left and right.

Miscellaneous excellent exercises

Overhead weight walks.

This is an excellent cardio exercise. You pick a bean, a heavy box or a dumbbell, and as you walk, you raise it. After a few steps, you bring it down and keep walking, raising and lowering the weight for a few minutes, depending on your body condition.

Sandbag/ bucket walk

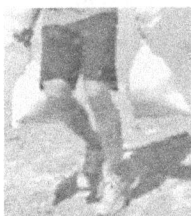

You pick up a kind of heavy bucket or sandbag, walk for a distance, and then, without stopping, change the bucket to the opposite arm. Breathe in and out without holding your breath. Again, depending on your physical condition, you decide how long to do it for. Excellent!

Crawling

Crawling is an excellent exercise, more than just something we did as babies; it's an integral part of who we are. It is the foundation. Learning how to crawl again can nourish your brain, tie your body together and remove physical barriers.

Crawling is a primitive pattern, or a developmental pattern, that we all have when we're born.

I sometimes practice crawling to the front and then backward. You can do it when you are on vacation, or when you don't have time to go to the gym or do cardio. Excellent Exercise.

Door Lat Pull

Hold on to the door handles to increase your grip. You can use a towel around the door, as shown. Stand as close to the door as possible. Squat your body as low as you can go, then pull yourself up toward the door, using only your arms. Concentrate on your lats. Perform as many reps as you can. Excellent back-lats exercise.

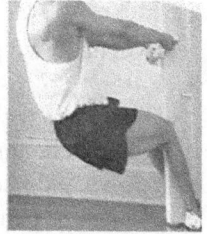

Striders

Bounce forward by pushing hard from the ball of your grounded foot, pumping your arms to generate speed. When you reach you target zone, turn around and comeback repeating the Strider to your starting position.

Skip

Bounce forward with your knees as high as you can, pump your arms to generate speed, reach your exercise zone, turn around and comeback. Skipping again.

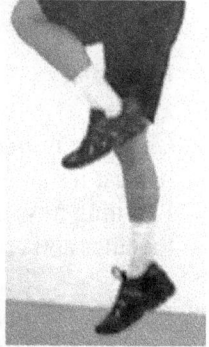

Plate push

Begin in all four in the push-up position with hands on the weight plate, driving the plate with drive forward, taking strikes as hard as possible for your goal distance.

Tire Exercises

Tire Flip

Squat low down, pick up the tire with both hands with an under grip. At the same time, stand up, pick the tire, change your hand position, and push and throw the tire forward. Repeat eight to ten reps.

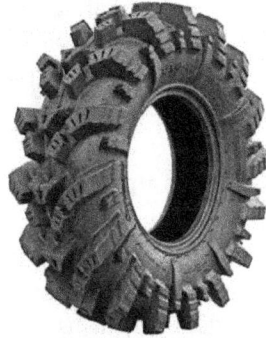

Overhead SledgeHammer Strike

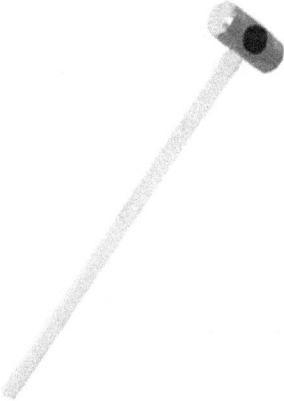

Grasp the SledgeHammer with both hands, position your hands appropriately if you are right-handed or left-handed, keep your feet shoulder apart, and from an over-the-shoulder overhead position, strike the tire, flexing your knees as you strike the tire.

Side SledgeHammer Strike

Begging with a wide stand, hold the hammer with hands far apart, strike the tire sideways. This action creates an action across the torso.

This is excellent exercise for the whole body, especially for the arms, shoulders, and chest. It is also excellent cardio-vascular exercise.

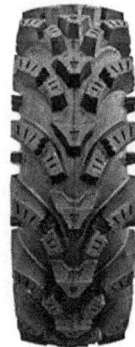

Medicine Ball

The medicine ball tones every muscle in your body and is excellent for your shoulders, arms, and entire body. Medicine balls range in weight from 10 to 40 pounds, and some even have a dual-grip handle.

Exercises:
Overhead squat

Overhead squats engage your core, your lower back. You're also working your upper back, shoulders, and arms.

Start by holding the medicine ball above your head with your feet shoulder-width apart. Hold the medicine ball straight over your head during the total movement.
Squat down: Begin to bend your knees as if you're going to sit in a chair.

Stop when your thighs are parallel to the ground. Push through your heels on the rise, giving your glutes a squeeze at the top.
Do 3 sets of 12 reps.

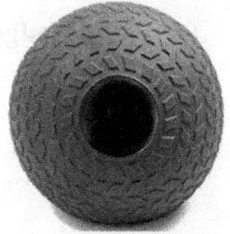

Circles

A fantastic shoulder exercise

Stand with your feet shoulder-width apart, holding the medicine ball straight overhead. Start to move your extended arms in a clockwise movement, making a circle from start to finish. You may twist your core to assist the exercise, but keep your feet stationary.

Do 8 to 10 reps in one direction, then change to doing another 8 to 10 reps in a counterclockwise direction.

Slams

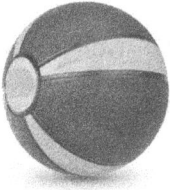

Used to develop power and strength, medicine ball slams are cardio work as well. If you have a heavier medicine ball available, this is the exercise to use it. Stand with your feet shoulder-width apart and the medicine ball straight above your head. Bend at your hips and, keeping your arms extended, slam the medicine ball into the ground as hard as you can. Pick up the medicine ball and return to the starting position. Do 3 sets of 10 reps.

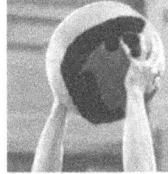

Shoulder press

Excellent for arms and shoulders.
Extend your arms to the ceiling, reaching the ball overhead, and then slowly lower the ball back to the starting position. Do 3 sets of 10 reps.

Biceps curl

Stand with your feet shoulder-width apart, holding the medicine ball in both hands at your chest. Keeping your elbows close to your body, lower the ball toward the ground until your arms are fully extended. Curl the ball back up to your chest. Lower the ball back to the starting position. Do 3 sets of 10 reps.

Wall pass

Find a medicine ball-safe wall. Stand 3 or 4 feet from the wall, holding a lightweight medicine ball with both hands, with feet shoulder width apart, keeping a slight bend in the knees and the core engaged. Bring the ball to your chest and throw it at the wall. Catch the ball on its return and repeat. Do 3 sets of 10 reps.

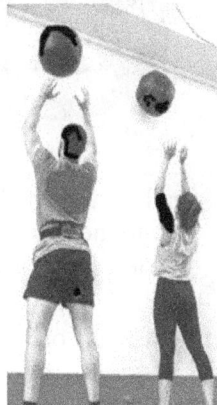

Medicine Ball Triceps Extension

This exercise builds arm and shoulder strength. The medicine ball triceps extension is an exercise similar to traditional arm extensions with dumbbells. From standing or seated, engage your abs and hold your spine upright.

Hold a medicine ball in both hands. Extend your arms overhead so they frame your ears. Bend your elbows, lowering the ball behind your head until your elbows form 90-degree angles.

Squeeze the triceps to straighten your arms, taking the ball back up again.

Do 3 sets of 10 reps.

Medicine Ball Diagonal Wood chops

The medicine ball diagonal wood chop is a vigorous exercise that strengthens the upper and lower body while targeting the abs and

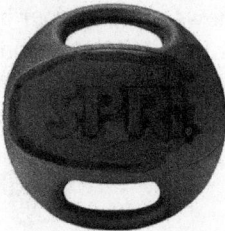

Obliques, the triceps, and the Lats. The shoulders will strengthen as the arms reach down and up.

Start with the feet shoulder apart and hold a medicine ball overhead at a diagonal toward the right side.

Step out to the left onto a lunge, pivoting the ball past the body toward the left side. Rotate the toe behind and also rotate the torso, taking the ball toward the back as far as you can. Step the left foot back to start while swinging the ball up and at a diagonal.

Do 3 sets of 10 reps each side.

Hammer workout

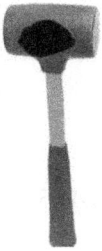

This is a complete shoulder, arm, and MMA strength conditioning program, especially for fighters that are throwing punches.

1- Swing the hammers from side to side at shoulder height behind and in front of your head, trying to archive a circle with the hammers.

2-Hold one hammer in front of you as you rotate the other one around your head.

3-Stand and imaging hitting the opponent with a hammer in a down-faction and overhead movement.

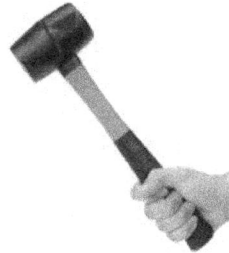

A SHORT HISTORY OF INDIAN CLUBS

Club swinging is credited with having been created in India to develop strength, balance, physical ability, and physical prowess in training soldiers; it has been used by wrestlers and martial artists for centuries. Their acceptance grew, and they were used in an Olympic sport in 1904, called "rhythmic gymnastics."
The United States Army Manual of Physical Training (1914) notes:

"The effect of these exercises, when performed with light clubs, is chiefly a neural one, hence they are primary factors in the development of grace, and coordination and rhythm. As they tend to supple the muscles and articulation of the shoulders and the upper and forearms and wrists, they are indicated in cases where there is a tendency toward what is ordinarily known as "muscle bound." (p.113).

In 1885, Baron Nils Posse, a Swedish soldier and physical professor, came to America and presented the Swedish system of medical and military gymnastics. I don't know for sure, but I believe the hammer workout replaced the Indian club along the way.

Poor exercises will cause injuries or force you to stop training for an extended period of time, if not indefinitely.

Here is a list of exercises that you must be very careful about doing.

1-Behind-the-Neck Shoulder Press:

It is good exercise for your shoulders, but bad for your joints. Be careful.

2-upright rows with a barbell:

It can be bad for your shoulder. Shoulder impingement happens when the tendon of the supraspinatus (a rotator cuff muscle) gets inflamed.

3-Twisting Sit-ups:

Many people do twisting sit-ups to target both the rectus abdominus (abs) and the obliques at the same time.

The problem is, spinal flexion puts a lot of pressure on the intervertebral discs.

4-Stiff-Legged Deadlifts with a Rounded Back:

Rounding your lower back puts a lot of undue stress on the nucleus pulposus of the discs. In addition to flexion, rotation also places more.Doing a stiff-legged deadlift with a rounded back is basically very unsafe; you are inviting a herniated disc!

That's why it's so imperative to protect your lower back all of the time. Keep your back flat during every movement, especially if there's added resistance involved. Constantly think, protect the low back-and you can't go wrong.

It is not enough to know your craft - you have to have feeling.
Édouard Manet

166

Train like a Fighter

Everybody wishes to gain muscle, lose fat, and be more athletic. Yet very few individuals can actually achieve that kind of body. Why? The reason is that most people are not willing to endure the time and effort it takes to obtain that kind of body. Fighters work out for strength, endurance, and mobility.

A fighter requires a body that's as powerful as it looks.

I used to think (and still think) that genetics is the reason why most power athletes have such incredible bodies.

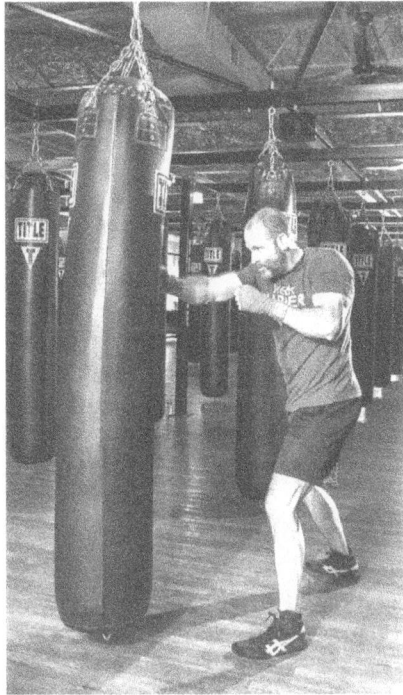

These guys make faster progress than anyone you'll ever see in the gym. After a few months of hard work, sweat, and incredibly hard workouts, they end up with a pretty damn impressive body. Also, I have seen the ones with poor genetics, with almost nothing to show after months of working out.

Here is strength, endurance, and mobility training you can do at the same time.

1-Pull-up as much as you can do-No rest
2-Push-up as much as you can do-No rest
3-Kettlebell squat with kettlebell or dumbbell thrust-No rest.
4: Forward/back/side-to-side running for a couple of minutes can be replaced by a skip rope—no rest.

5-Punching Bag –uppercuts-jabs-Heavy Punching-No Rest for 15 seconds and repeat the sequence four more times.

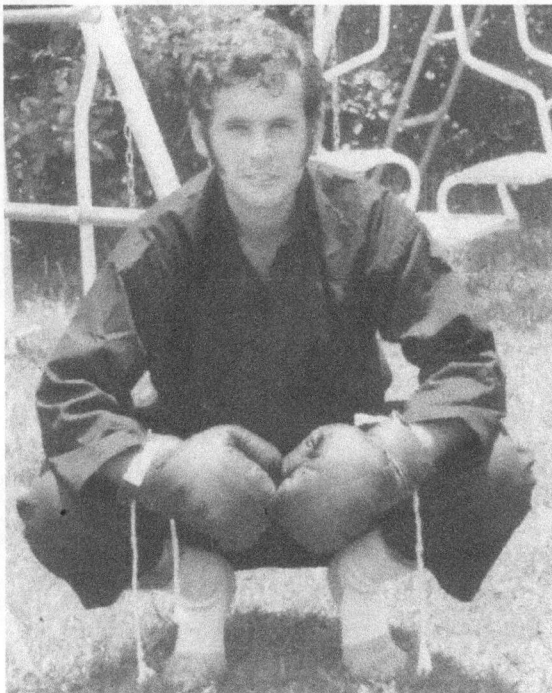

The Author Practicing 50 years ago

This kind of training demonstrates the importance of constantly moving, just like a fighter.

Start training to develop strength, endurance, and mobility, and you may obtain a fighter body,

It is going to take time, months, but if you keep it up, you will look fantastic.

My advice is to stop doing traditional cardio exercises on a treadmill or a bike. Instead, jump rope, do sprints, do fast walks. You'll get leaner, stronger, and more mobile. Training like a fighter insures that you'll build strength, endurance, and mobility at the same time. This is not everything you do in a workout, but if you do it for a couple of months, adding more sets, you work out your entire body. Just like a fighter.

Start training your body to move better and you'll end up looking better.

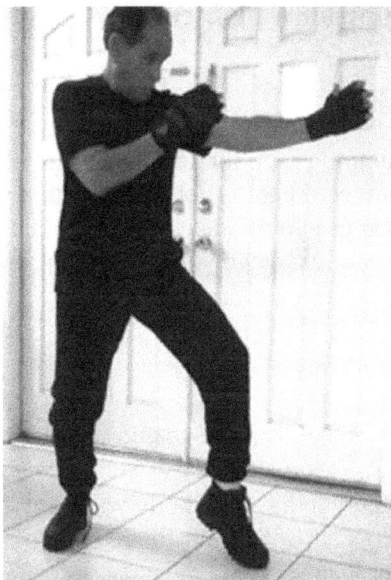

One of the best tips I can give you is to stop doing so many of the usual cardio exercises on a treadmill or bike.

As a substitute, work with a few circuits per week like the one I outlined above.

You'll get leaner, stronger, and more mobile.

The Author still practices every day in 2023.

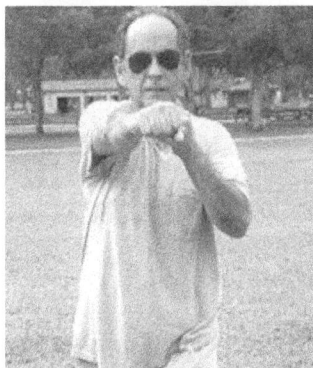

Frank Marchante practicing martial arts very early in the morning. (2023)

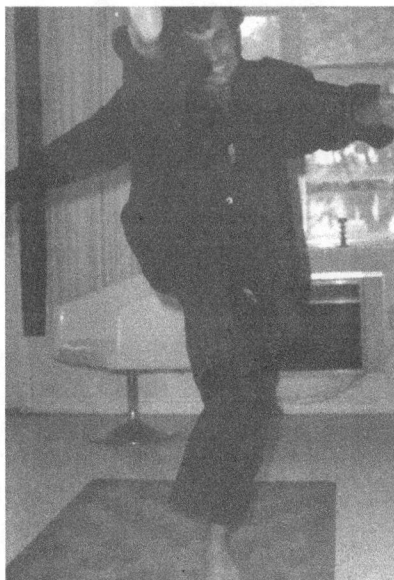

The Author, practicing the front kick 50 years ago

Jumping Rope for a Fighter body

The muscles you use while jumping rope for 15 minutes are like those used when running for 30 minutes. There is not a muscle that you don't use in jumping rope. You use your hands, wrists, shoulders, and every part of your legs, from your calves to your thighs, and the constant movement works your heart and lungs.

1. Diet When You Need

You shouldn't diet; you should make lifestyle changes.

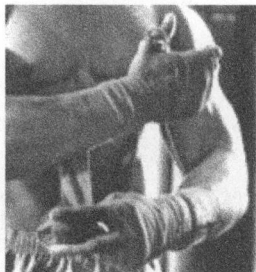

When you have the body you want, then follow a healthy nutritional plan to maintain your leanness.

Losing fat quickly demands an attitude toward eating that can't be maintained throughout your life.

You go on a diet when you need to make significant body composition changes in a short amount of time, like a special situation, wedding, competition, ECT.

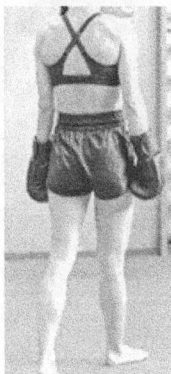

2. Because it sounds really good doesn't mean it's good

Make a smart choice; don't believe everything you hear. There many gimmick apparatus and diets out there. Many are good, and many are not.

Research yourself what people have experienced from diets and gym equipment. Read, research, talk to people and find out their experience. Don't just believe advertisement.

3. Focus on your workouts

People are always asking, How long should I work out? How many reps/how many sets? How many days a week? Concentrate on a good workout. It doesn't matter if it's short or long.

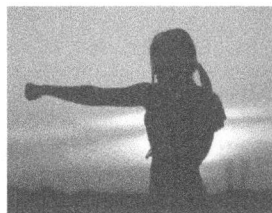

If you are trying to bulk up, shorter and heavier is the key. I've never taken 2-4 minute rest periods. My workouts never last long because I have always used short rest periods. Make sure to focus on the muscle you are working with each rep. Do two compound exercises.

Keep the rest periods short and you will be on your way to better shape. Why are people so worried about how many reps, sets, or time they have at the gym? Focus on getting a good workout.

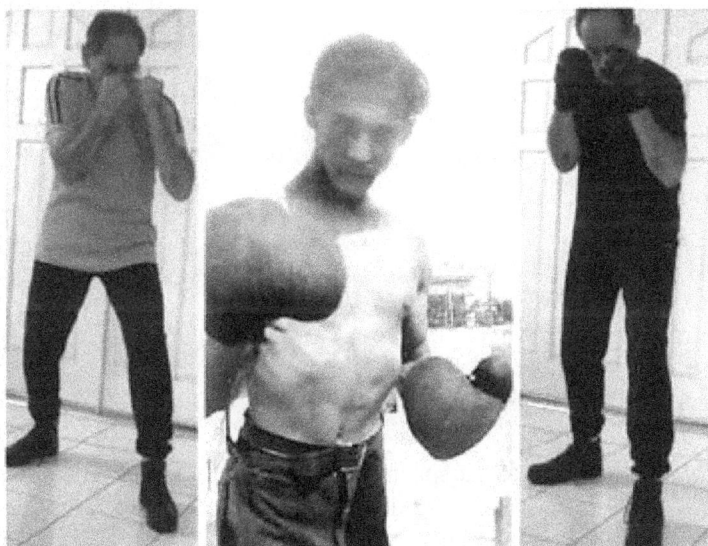

The author is pictured with his father in the center, who taught him how to defend himself at a very young age, the same thing he did with his son years later

Sprint Training

Purchase good running shoes, preferably medium-high ones, to protect your ankles.

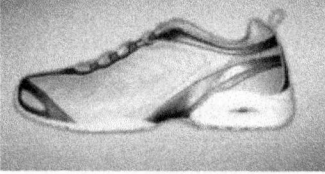

Star with a 3-minute warm up walk. This will make you breathe a bit hard and deeper. This is because you are working on your heart and lungs.

Sprint as hard as you can to a nearby spot. When you reach that point, stop, and walk back breathing slowly.

Here you are trying to slow down your breathing and your heart. Start with one sprint and, as you progress and get used to sprinting, try to do 4 or 5 sprints, trying to run faster as you progress.

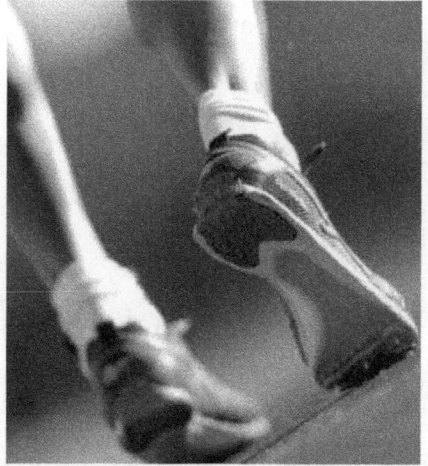

Sprint, walk back, sprint, walk back, spring, walk back. Look over the ground where you are going to sprint for holes in the ground or rocks so you don't hurt your ankles.

The theory learned that sprinters had strong looking bodies, strong legs and calves, while long-distance runners had very skinny, non-muscular looking bodies.

So Arthur, Mike and Vince said the trick is to do short, hard workouts. They said you **"can't train hard for too long"**. It is either short and hard or long and easier.

Arthur and Mike also said you had to rest 2 to 3 days in between exercise days. I personally follow this plan. You know? It works perfectly not only for me but for many others.

Always cool down, walk around, swing your arms, move your body, shake your legs, and then do your stretching exercises.

You have plenty of options to do this kind of training. Stair climbing, cliff sprinting, running in place, you can even use this system while riding a bicycle or sprinting up a small hill.

Believe me, this type of training will help you lose body fat while also building muscle and strength in your legs and calves. Your belly fat and spare tire will vanish as if by magic.

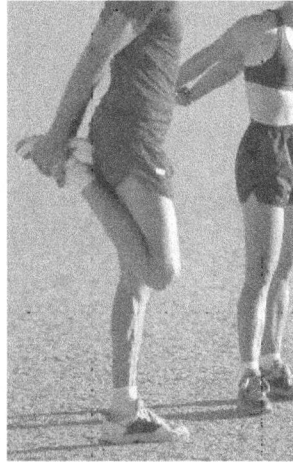

You are also getting a great heart and lung workout at the same time.

If you are a female, you will be developing a shape that you could only dream about. Toned, healthy, muscled, trim and lean, for men and women will be the outcome.

Never be so arrogant that you fail to give people the benefit of being as stupid as they actually are.

Arthur Jones

Free Exercise Routine-Woman

Arms

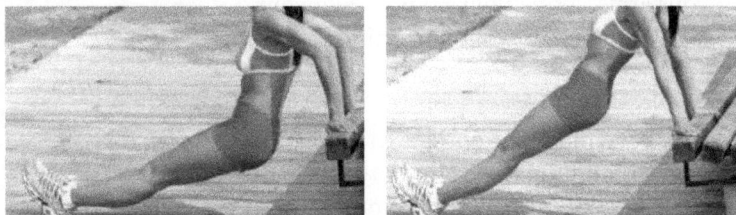

Triceps Dips 3 sets /8 reps

Chest/arms

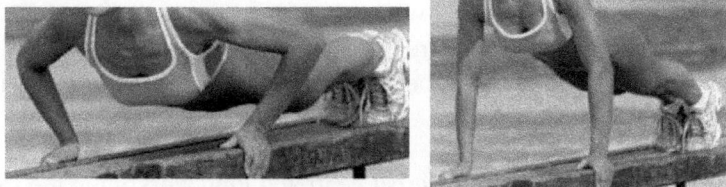

Push-ups 3 sets /8 reps

Push-ups

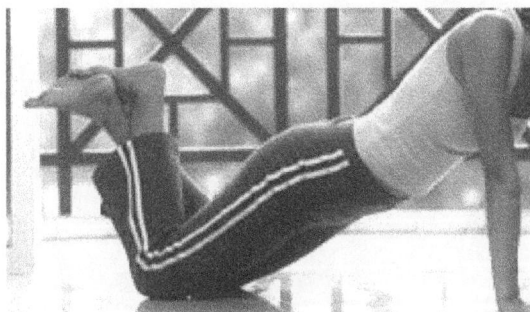

Push-ups (if you can't do regular Push-ups yet)

Abdomen

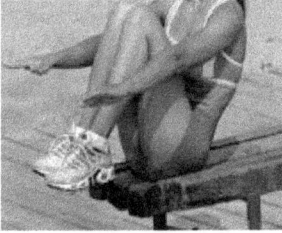
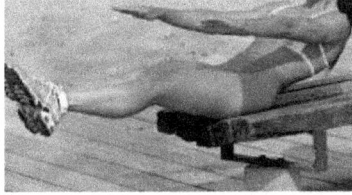

Knees Raises 3 sets /8 reps

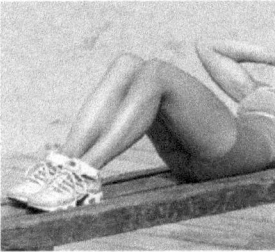
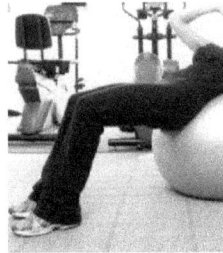

Crunches 3 sets /8 reps   **Sit-ups** 3 sets /8 reps

Cardio

Depends in
Shape

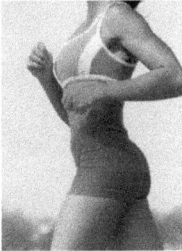
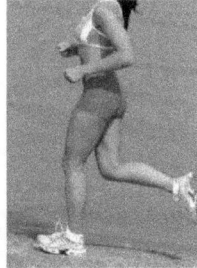

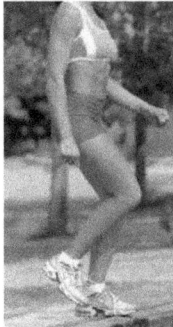

Steps -up
3 sets /8 reps

Woman Basic Routines

Lose body fat and gain muscle with three workouts a week.

Warm-up

Dumbbells swing, or treadmill walking.
Toe touching

Abdomen

Crunches sit-ups   3sets/8 reps
Kneeling back kicks 3sets/8 reps

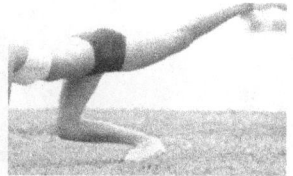

Kneeling back kicks

Chest/Pecs

Bench press
3 sets/8 reps
Flyes/peck deck
3 sets/8 reps

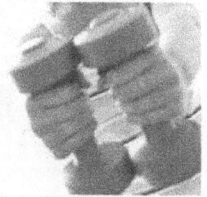

Shoulders

Lateral raises
3 sets/8reps
Dumbbell Front raises
3 sets/8 reps

Dumbbell Front raises

Back

Barbell / Dumbbell rows 3 sets/8 reps

Arms

Barbell/Dumbbell Curls	3sets/ 8 reps
Triceps press down	3sets/ 8 reps

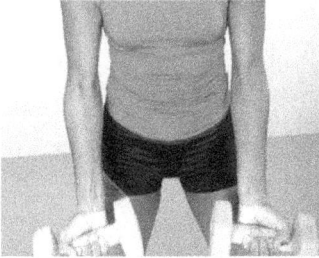 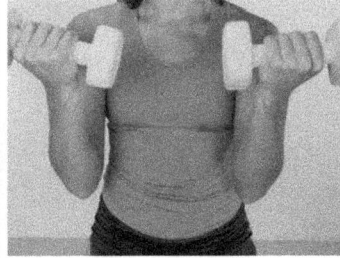

Dum bbell Curls

Legs/thighs

Hack Squat	3sets/8 reps
Leg extensions	3sets/8 reps

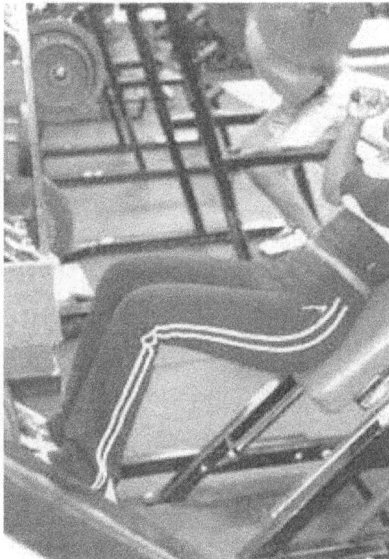

Hack Squat

Calves

Toe Raises   3 sets /8reps

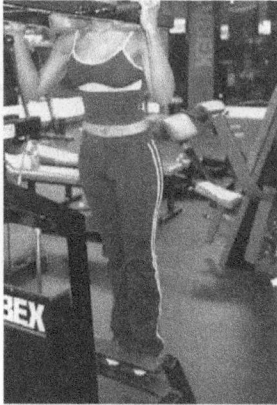 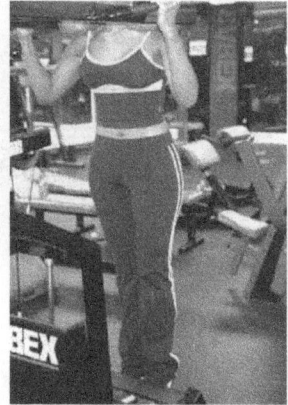

Start   Finished

Aerobic exercises are done on the same days or even better, on alternate days. After 3 months, you can move to the intermediate routine.

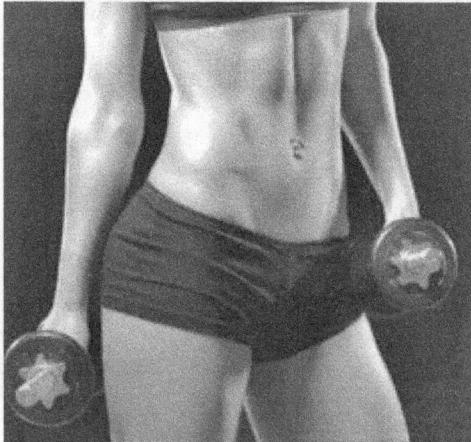

Throw caution to the wind and just do it.
Carrie Underwood

Intermediate/advance routine

Warm-up

Dumbbells swing, treadmill walking

Abdomen (not shown)

Crunches sit-ups	3 sets/8 reps
Side leg kicks	3 sets/8 reps
Kneeling back kicks	3 sets/8 reps

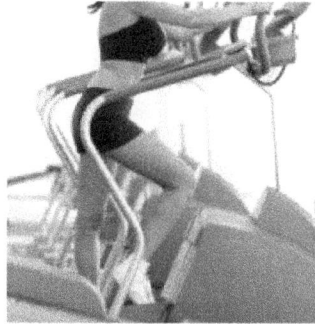

Chest/pecs

Bench press	3 sets/8reps
Flyes/ peck deck	3 sets/8 reps

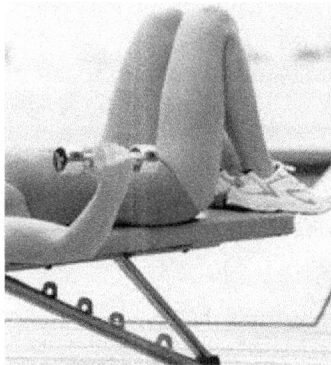

Flyes

Shoulders

Dumbbell Lateral raises	3 sets/8reps
Dumbbell Front raises	3 sets/8 reps
Barbell Press	3 sets/8reps
Bent over Laterals raises	3 sets/8reps
Dumbbell press	3 sets/8reps

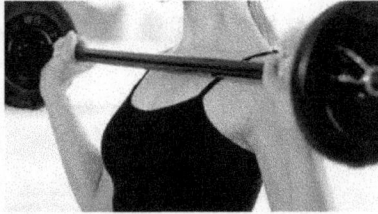

Barbell Press

Dumbbell Lateral raises

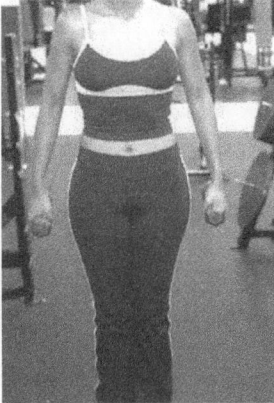

Start

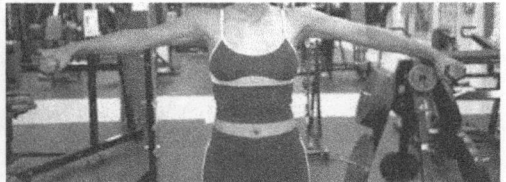

Finished

Arms

Barbell /dumbbell curls	3 sets/ 8 reps
Preacher Curls	3 sets/ 8 reps
Lat Triceps pushdown	3 sets/ 8 reps

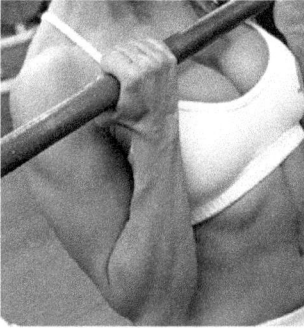

Start

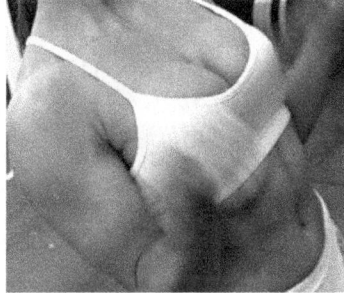

Barbell curls

Finished

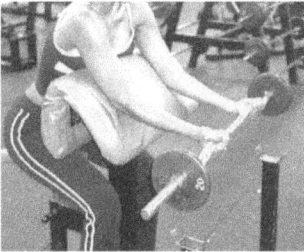 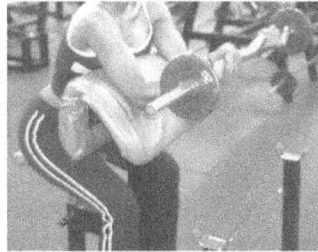

Start   Finished

Preacher Curls

Triceps pushdown

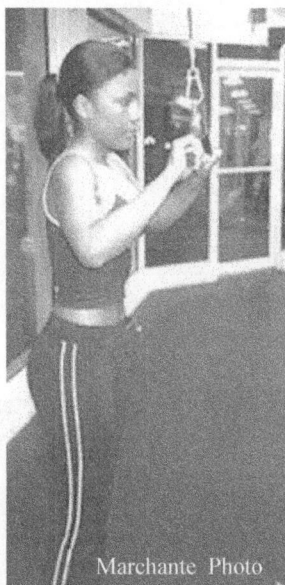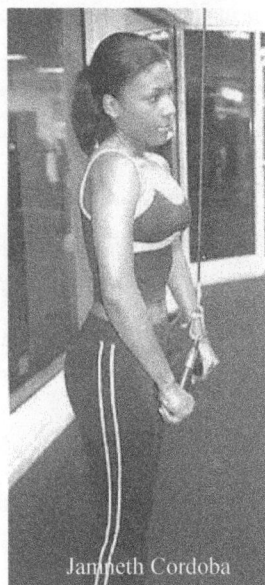

Marchante Photo   Janneth Cordoba

   Start   Finished

Woman arms

This area is one of the biggest problems for women; they accumulate excess fat in this area. Remember, there is no spot reducing. Aerobics will reduce fat in the whole body, not just in one area.

There are two muscle groups in the upper arms: the triceps and the biceps. The triceps run through the arm from the shoulder to the elbow, and the biceps run from the front of the shoulder to the inside of the elbow. You extend the arm and push with the triceps; the biceps flex the arm to work as a lifting muscle.

Back

Dumbbells rows	3 sets/8reps
Barbell/machine rows	3 sets/8reps

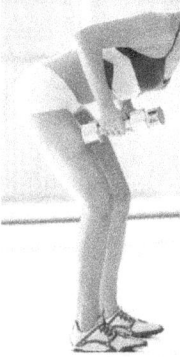
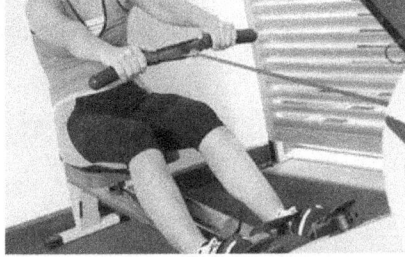

Dumbbells rows   Machine/ Barbell Rows

Legs

Hack Squats	3sets/8 reps
Leg extensions	3sets/8 reps
Leg press	3sets/8 reps
Lunges	3sets/8 reps

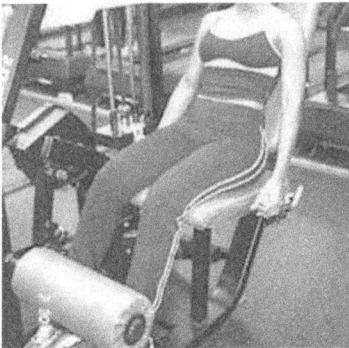
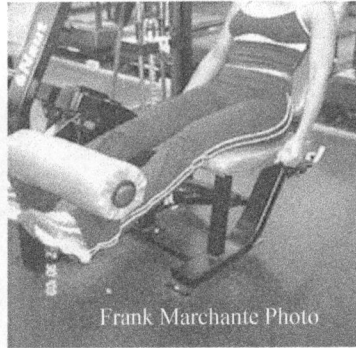

Legs Extensions

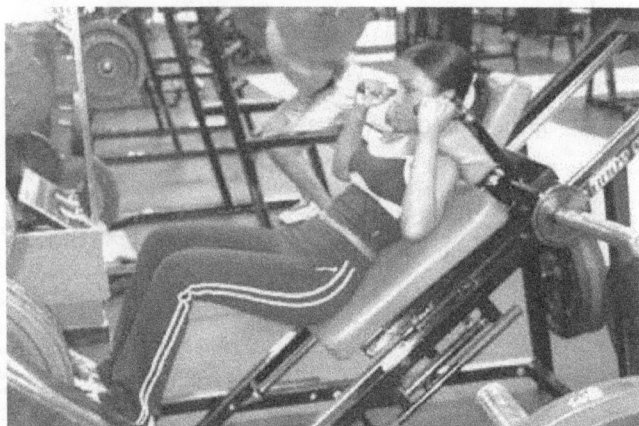

Hack Squats

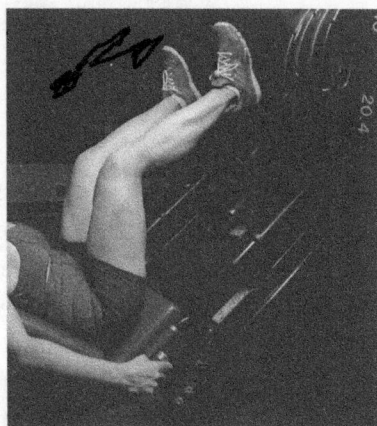

Leg Press

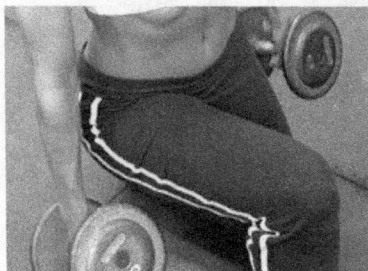

Lunges

Calves

Standing Toe Raises 3 sets /8reps
Seated toe raises   3 sets / 8 reps

Standing calves raises

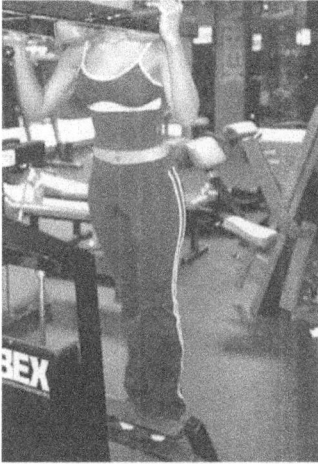 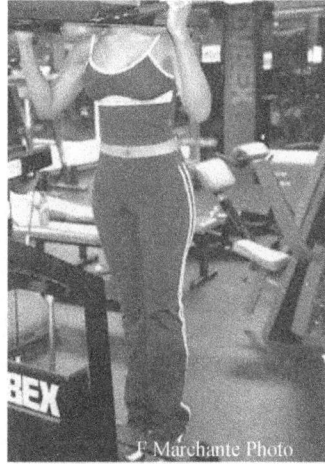

Start   Finished

Aerobic exercises are done on the same day or every other day. At this point, you can also use a split routine.

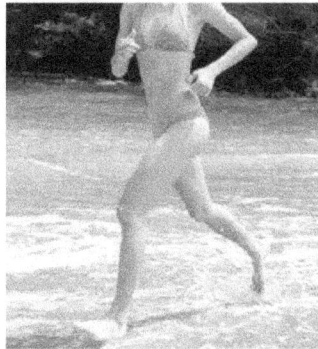

Advance woman Routine workout

Warm-up

Dumbbells swing, treadmill walking.
Toe touching

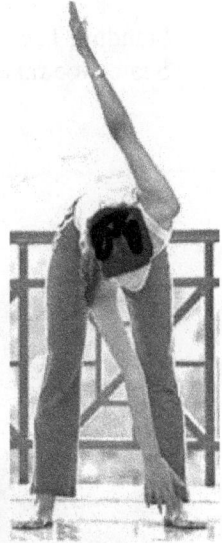

Abdomen

Alternating knees touch   3 sets /8 reps
Sit-ups/ on ball   3 sets /8 reps

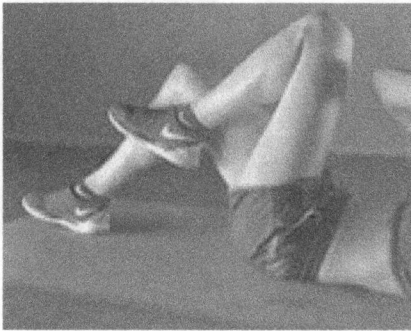

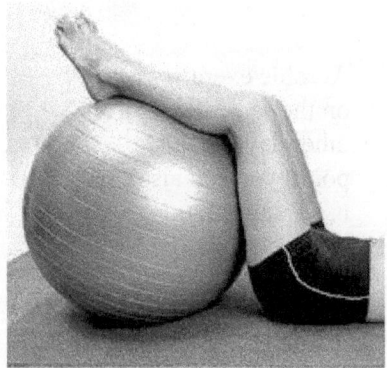

Abdomen (continuation)

Crunches sit-ups	3 sets /8 reps
Kneeling back kicks	3 sets/8 reps
Knees Raises	3 sets/8 reps

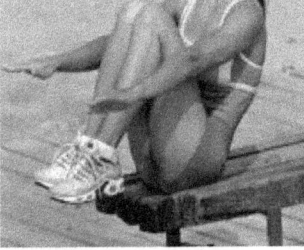 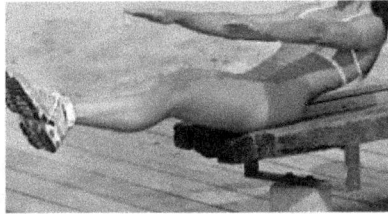

Chest

Bench press	4 sets/8reps
Flyes/ peck deck	4 sets/8reps
Dumbbell Pullover	4 sets /8reps

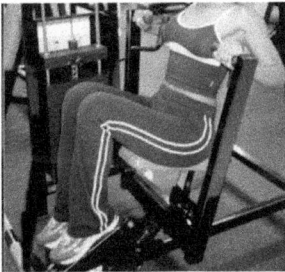 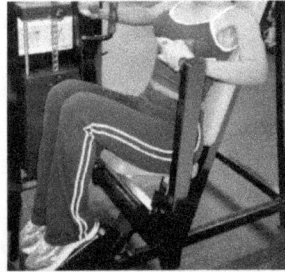

Bench Press

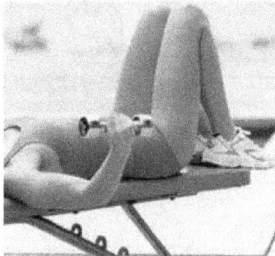

Flys

Shoulders

Dumbbell Lateral raises	4 sets/8reps
Dumbbell Front raises	4 sets/8 reps
Bent over Laterals raises	4 sets/8 reps
Barbell/Dumbbell Press	4 sets/8 reps

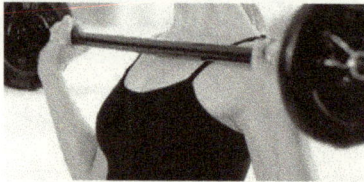

Barbell Shoulder Press

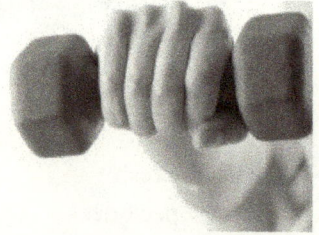

Dumbbell Front Raises

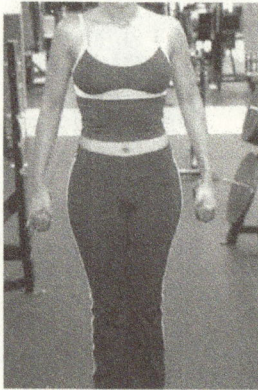

Start

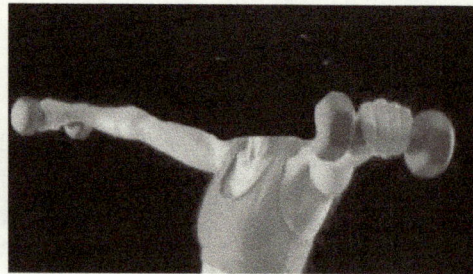

Finished

Dumbbell Lateral raises

Back

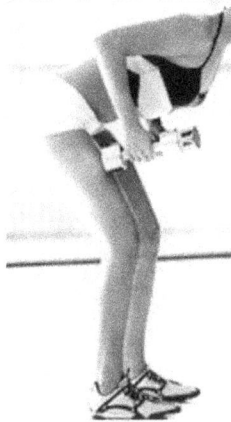

Dumbbells rows   4 sets /8reps
Barbell rows/ machine 4 sets/ 8 reps
Lat Pulley-front/back   4sets/8 reps

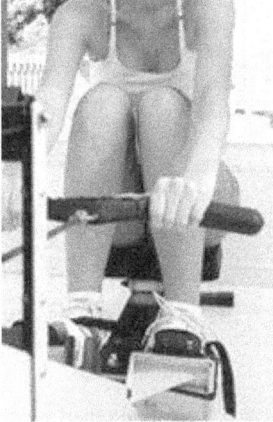

Rows   Dumbbells rows

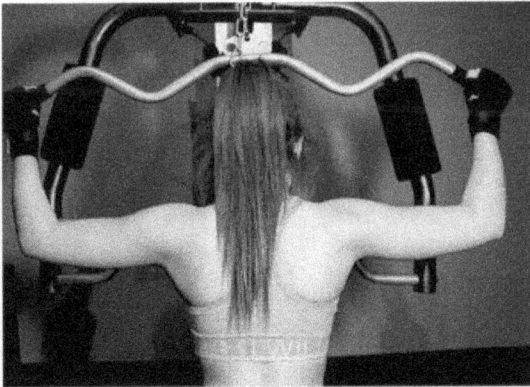

Lat Pulley pull down to the front/back

189

Arms

Barbell /dumbbell curls	3 sets/ 8 reps
Preacher Curls	3 sets/ 8 reps
Lat Triceps pushdown	3 sets/ 8 reps

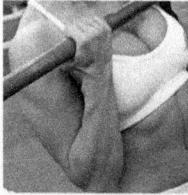

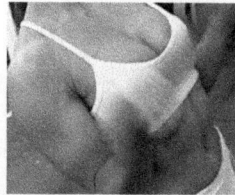

Barbell curls

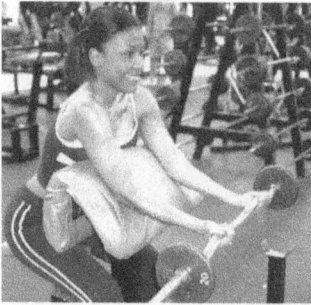

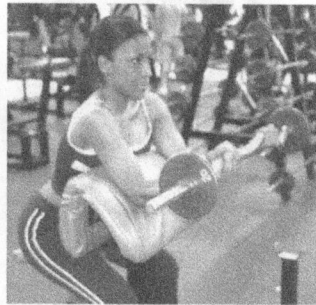

Preacher Curls

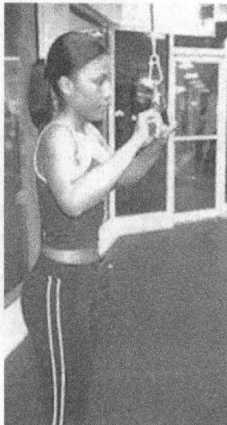

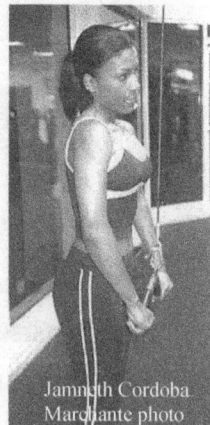

Jamnath Cordoba
Marchante photo

Triceps push down

Legs

Leg extensions	4 sets /8 reps
Hack Squats	4 sets/8 reps
Leg press	4 sets /8 reps
Lunges	4 sets/8 reps

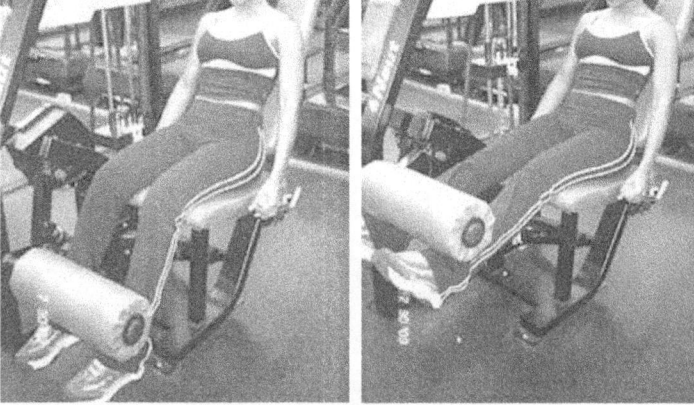

Leg extensions

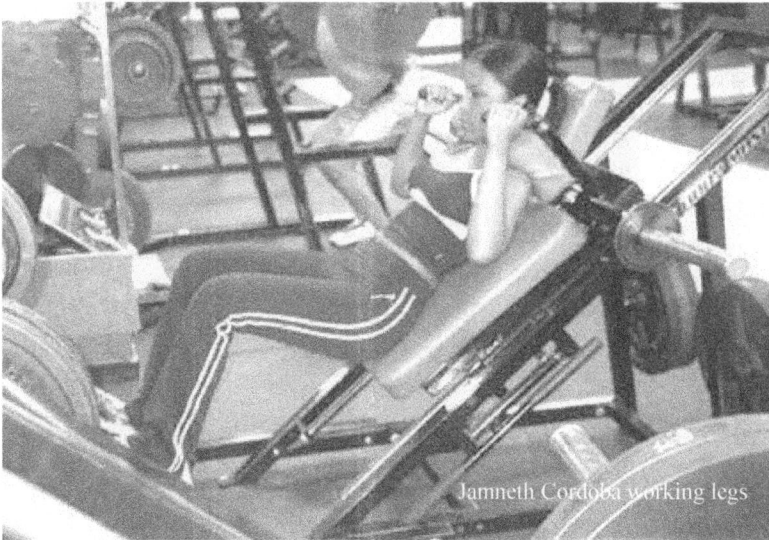

Hack Squats

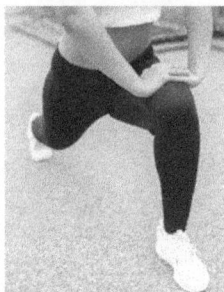
Lunges

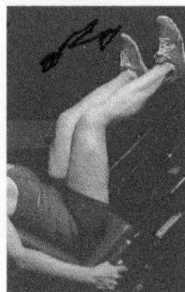
Leg press

Calves
Standing Toe Raises   3 sets /8reps
Seated toe raises   3 sets / 8 reps

Standing calves raises

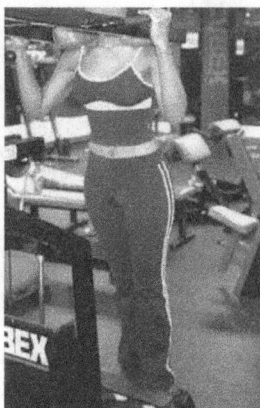
Start

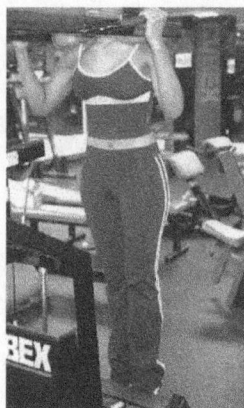
Finished

Aerobic exercises are done on alternate days. At this point, you can also use a split routine.

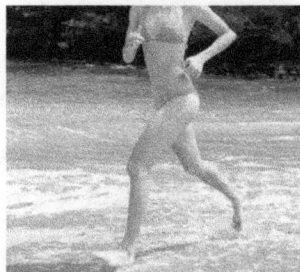

Strong and healthy is the new sexy.
Ronda Rousey

Cardio Explanation

You lower your growth hormone when cardio is done before weights, limiting muscle growth and strength when hitting the weights. Do cardio after weight training or another day. A three-minute warm-up at a slow pace on a tread-mill is all you need for a warm-up. **Stay away** from cardio in a bulk mass phase; do it only for a very short time as a warm-up.

Cardio to lose weight

When there is glycogen available for fuel, your body won't tap into your body fat stores. That is why you never want to eat or drink any carbohydrates before cardio. The first cardio should be done when you wake up on an empty stomach or at least two hours after eating, when there are no glycogen stores in your muscles if your goal is to lose fat and get hard. Fat burning is greatest during the first 15 minutes.

Ways to Burn Fat at Home

1. Chopping Wood
2. Push Mowing the Lawn
3. Shoveling Snow by Hand
4. Moving Furniture
5. Heavy House Cleaning
6. Painting the House
7. Weeding
8. Light House Cleaning
9. Washing the Windows
10. Gardening

Men Beginners Workout

This Program is brief and to the point

3 sets-8 reps each /3 times a week

Barbell – Machine
Chest
3x8 Bench Press
3x8 Flyes/peck

Barbell–Machine
Back
3x8 Dumbbell Row Motion
3x8 Lat Pulldown to the front
3x8 Chin to the Front

Barbell–Machine
Shoulder
3x8 Lateral Raises
3x8 Presses behind Neck

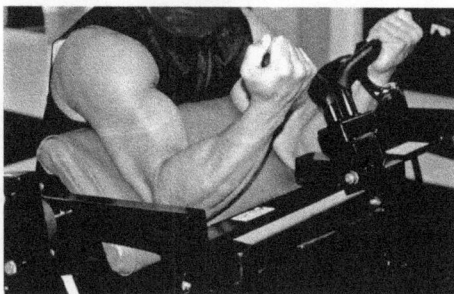

Arms-Barbell–Machine
3x8 Standing Barbell Curl
3x8 Lying Triceps Barbell Extension
3x8 Preacher Curl
3x8 Press Down on Lat Machine

Legs
3x8 Squats
3x8 Leg Extensions

Calves
3x8 Seated Calf Raises

BACK

A mighty back is a must for a weight lifter as well as a bodybuilder. To me, a big, wide, V-tapered back means a strong back. A back that does not have well-developed trapezius muscles is not a strong, wide-looking back.

The muscles in the back are called rhomboids, trapezius (traps), and latissimus dorsi. Lats are the second largest muscles in the body.

Some people, such as Steve Reeves, did not exercise the trapezius muscles.

Some claimed that developing the trapezius muscles would take away from your tapered or V-shaped appearance; others did not agree with that. What do you think?

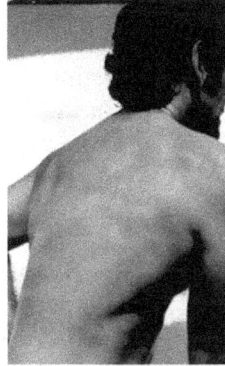

Author back younger years

The job of the trapezius muscles is to erect your body, and the latissimus dorsi (lats) are to widen the shoulders; people call the lats "wings".

The deltoids (deltoid is a word that originated from the Greeks) are muscles that gap the shoulders in a way that is somehow related to the back. There are also the spinal erectors, which are located at each side of the spine from the neck to the pelvis.

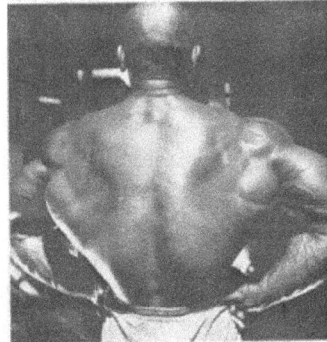

Sergio Oliva back by Denie

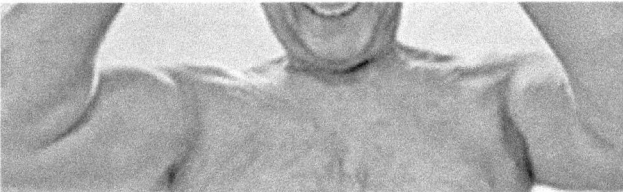

Frank Marchante -2023

Back

One of the advantages
of the one-arm
dumbbell row is the
ability to protect your
lower back. With one
hand resting on a
bench or low table,
it takes the stress off
your lower back.

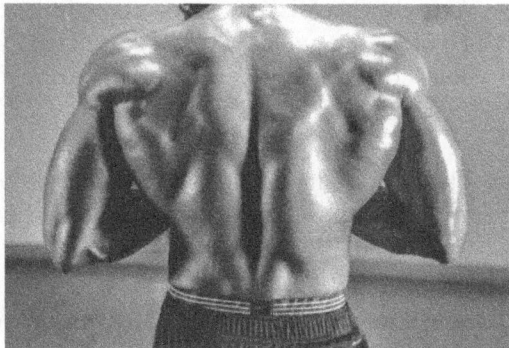

If your gym does not
have a T-bar machine, just take a barbell and load the plates to one
side and stick the other corner of the bar into a corner. Keep your
hand closed to the plates and do one set with your right hand touching
the plates, and then do another set with your left hand touching the
plates.

Arthur Jones and champion Mike
Mentzer came to the conclusion
that you can't train hard for a long
period, just like a sprinter can run
at top speed for a long distance.

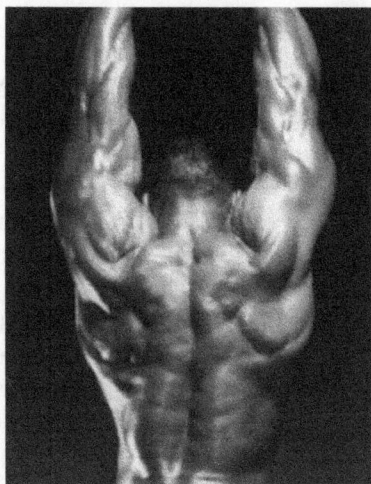

Arthur Jones believed that you do
not need more than 2 sets of any
exercise. Mike adapted his ideas.

If you continue using the same
weight and same repetitions for
too long, you will not progress.
After some time, you will reach a
sticking point.

Sergio Oliva back

Intermediate/Advance routine

Along with squats, I think the deadlift is one of the best all-around exercises. Bend your knees, then grasp a barbell with a slighter shoulder width, using an under/over grip. One palm faces down, the other faces up. Keep your back flat and your head up. Stand up straight with no jerking or pulling, until your body is perpendicular to the ground, pause, and lower the bar under control.

Back
Deadlift 3x8 reps.

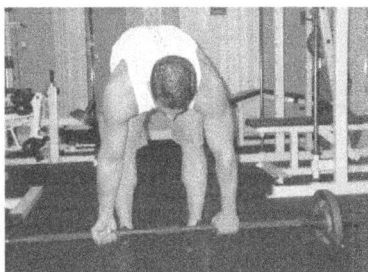

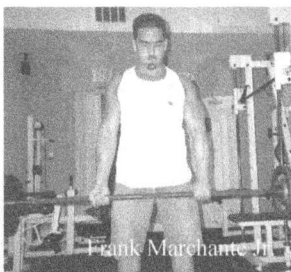

Palm–up Pull downs – (not shown) Grap the bar with the palms-up grip. Most people use the palm-down grip. Pull the bar from overhead into the chest around upper pec area, hold and return slowly to top. 3x8 reps.

Barbell Rows - It's the most popular and effective exercise for developing the back. You can do it with a barbell, machine or dumbbell. Stand close to the bar; bend over at waist, parallel to floor with head up; row the bar up to the lowest part of your chest; lower the bar and without touching the floor. 3x8 reps.

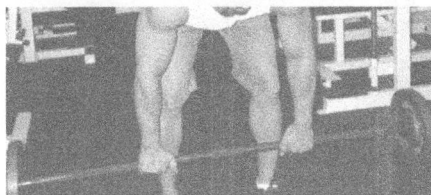

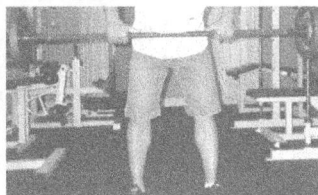

Rowing Machine - Sitting on the machine seat, grasp the handles and row. Contract, pause for a second or two, and let go. There are many ways to do this. There are different rowing machines, but all of them are similar and the concepts are the same. This is a good latissimus exercise. 3x8 reps.

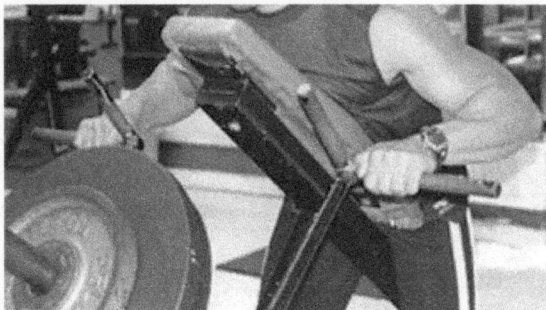

Frank Marchante Jr.

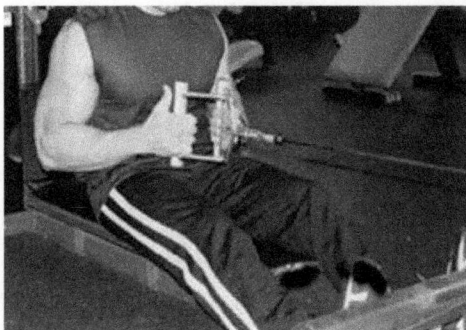

Frank Marchante Jr

Low Pulley Rowing- Place the feet against the machine. Pull the cable toward your mid-section. Stretch your lats while keeping your arms straight at the start of the movement. Good mid-back exercise. 3x8 reps.

Wide Grip Chin to the Front - Excellent for making your back wide. Hang from a chin bar using a wide overhand grip. Place your feet behind your knees so they won't touch the floor and pull

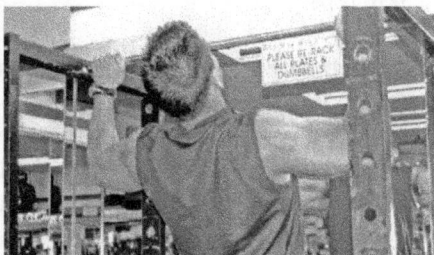

yourself up until your chin is over the bar. Lower yourself under control to the beginning position. 3x8 reps.

One Arms Dumbbell Rows - One-arm dumbbells rows are performed in the same manner as barbells rows. Keep your free hand resting on the bench for support, taking the stress out of your low back.

Raise the dumbbell as high as you can, a little bit above your torso, and pause for a second or two. Lower the dumbbell all the way down and get a good stretch at the end. Excellent for the lats. 3x8 reps.

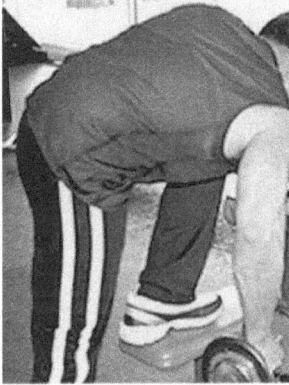

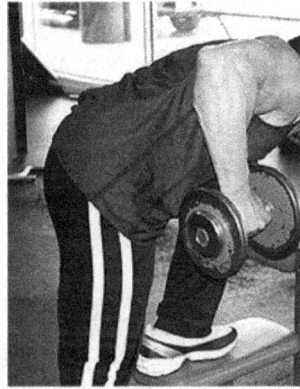

Photos F.Marchante

T-bar Rowing- It is done in a similar way to barbell rowing. With one end of the bar anchored to the floor. Some people prefer to stand on a block to keep the plates from hitting the floor and preventing getting a good stretch.

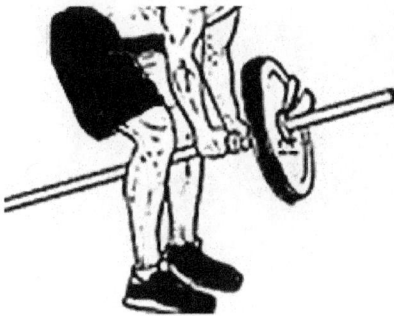

Grasp the bar with one hand on top of each other or next to each other. And bring the plates close to your chest.

This is a tremendous exercise for the latissimus, but also good for the rear deltoids. 3x8 reps.

Lat Machine pulls down to the front
Sit under the pulley, take a wide grip on the Lat machine bar, and pull down to the chest.

Let the weight take your arms back to full length. 3x8 reps.

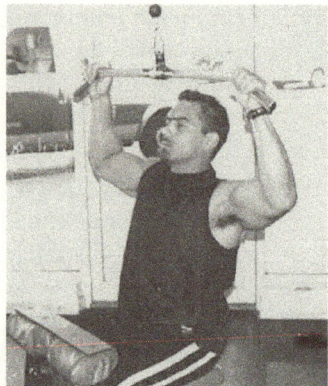

Dumbbell Pullovers It can be done on a decline or flat bench. It is good for the upper and lower chest. Also good for the lats. Lie flat on a flat bench with your feet flat on the floor. Holding dumbbells in a straight arm position, lower the dumbbells all the way back past your head as you inhale, pause a second or two, and then return the dumbbells back up as you exhale. 3x8 reps.

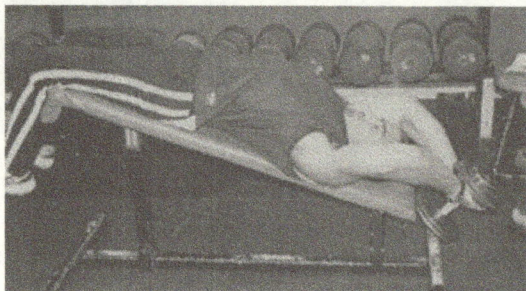

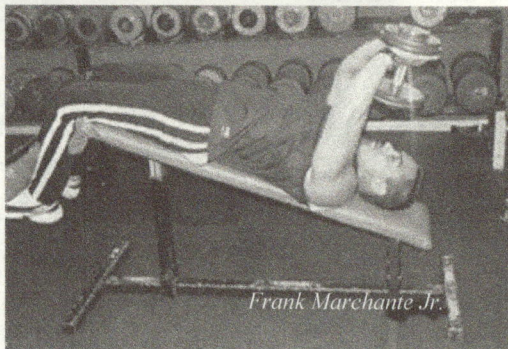

Frank Marchante Jr.

Chest

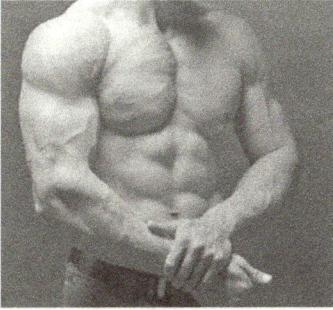

The pectoralis major (Latin origin) muscles cover each half of your front chest. These muscles turn your arms inward and pull your arms forward and down.

The pectoralis minor is located under your pectoralis major. It helps keep your shoulder blades down.

Pecs is the word used when referring to these muscles. In addition to developing these muscles, the serratus anterior muscles should be developed too. What you are trying to accomplish here is to develop your pecs. You want to add muscle where it belongs, not have pecs that hang or look like a woman's breasts when you're not wearing a shirt.

You are after square, sculpturing pecs, and must develop your upper and lower pecs. Incline exercises work the upper pecs and decline exercises work most of your lower pecs. Stretch and flex your pecs between sets.

Bench Press: Use a wide grip, holding the barbell at arm's length, lowering the bar with elbows away from the body until it touches your upper chest or neck. Inhale on the way down, exhale on the way up. The best exercise to pack a massive upper body.

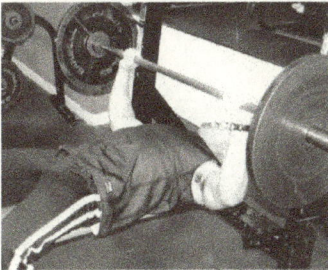

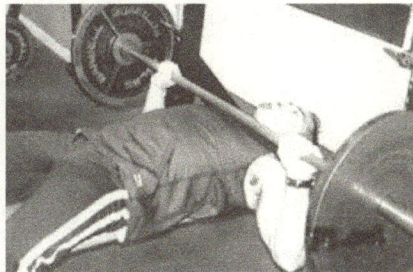

Frank Marchante Jr

201

Parallel Dip- Place your Chin against your chest, and slightly round your back. Lower your body down and rise up to a straight arm position, lower and rise continuously.

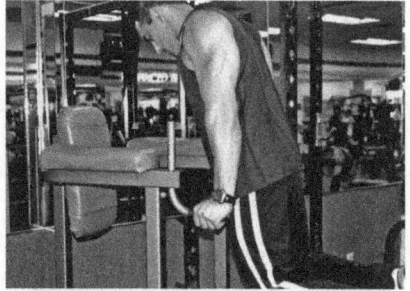

Narrow dips with elbows close in will promote triceps development; wide dips will target the chest. This is a great exercise for the pecs and also for the deltoids too.3x8reps.

Breathing Pullover - Breathing pullovers are done after heavy squats. It's mostly an exercise for the back, but is also expands the thorax and enlarges your rib cage. It also hits the upper chest and the lower chest.

It can be done with a barbell or a dumbbell on a flat bench, across a flat bench or decline bench. Do not use too much weight here. Lying down on a flat bench using dumbbells or a barbell at arm's lengths, bring it back over your head with arms almost straight all the way back, inhaling deep and exhaling when bringing arms up. 3x8 reps.

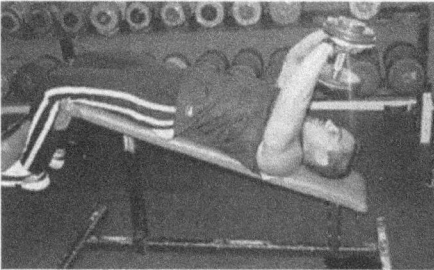

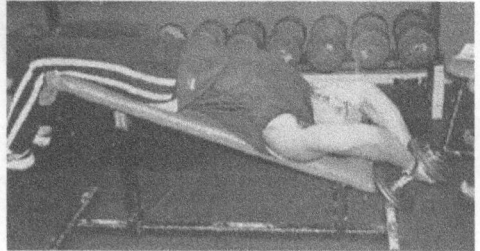

Peck Deck - Sit in position with your forearms against the machine pads. Push both pads at once all the way to where the arms meet, pause in this contracted position, and bring the arms back in a controlled way to the staring position. This is one of the best pectoral exercises.3x8 reps

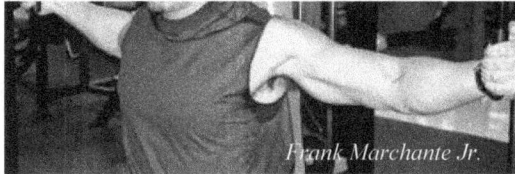

Frank Marchante Jr.

Barbell Incline Press - Sitting on a bench and holding a barbell in front of your chest by your lower pecs. Press upwards to arms lengths and bring it back under control. Excellent for pecks, front and side deltoid. 3x8 reps.

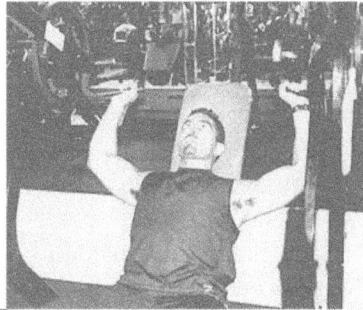

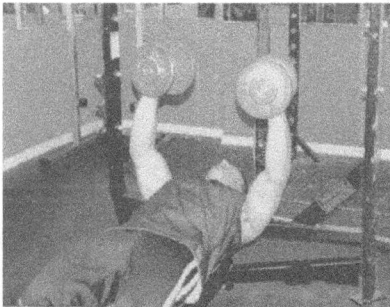

Flys Lie face up on a flat bench with a dumbbell in each hand, lifting the dumbbells to hold them directly over the chest. Press them up so the arms are extended (but not locked) over the center of the chest, with palms facing in to start.

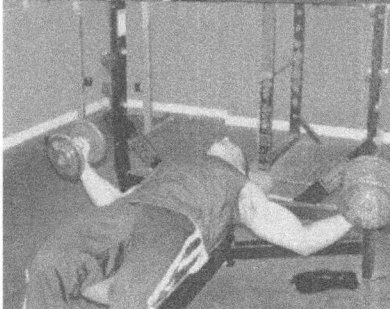

Keeping your elbows slightly bent, inhale and slowly lower both arms out to the sides while your shoulder blades naturally retract. Pause when the dumbbells reach shoulder height. 3x8 reps

SHOULDERS

The deltoids have 3 heads: front, lateral, and posterior. To accomplish this goal, all of them must be developed. Shoulder width is hereditary, but this does not mean you cannot acquire a nice pair of wide Delts if you work on them. The Deltoids (delts) help raise your arms forward, sideways, and backwards. The rotator cuff muscles lift and turn your arms.

The trapezius muscles lie over your shoulders and back. Their function is to help raise your shoulders.

Multiple studies have shown that women rate broad shoulders as one of the most attractive features of a man's physique.

Traps/shoulders

Many champions, including me, believe that having smaller traps will make your shoulders look square and broader. Thick trapezius development gives you the appearance of narrow, wide shoulders.

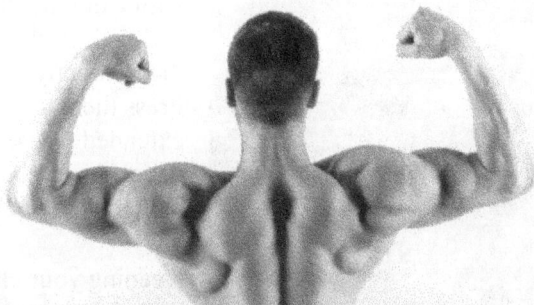

When I work my shoulders, I like to do presses and lateral raises to the front, sides, and back. You have to attack your delts with brutal intensity, isolating the three heads, pumping them so hard you cannot even raise your arms at the end of your workout. You are after massive, outstanding, humongous, muscular, and wide shoulders, and you are not going to get them by being soft or doing light-weight exercises.

Think wide, train hard, exercise the three heads, isolate the muscles, and workout with determination, and soon you will have terrific, powerful, wide-looking shoulders that will make you stand out from the rest with pride. Let's start working.

Press Behind Neck-This one works all three Delts' heads, the upper back, the trapezius, and, to some degree, the triceps. Perform this exercise in a slow way. Take a barbell with a shoulder-width grip and, keeping the elbows to the sides, lower the bar behind your neck. As soon as it touches your neck, bring it to arm's length.
Many people claim this kind of exercise, along with chins up and pulling down behind the neck, causes rotator cuff damage. All of these exercises are just as good when performed from the front. Keep this in mind if you have rotator cuff damage. 3x8 reps.

Dumbbells Front Raises - Place a pair of dumbbells in front of your thighs. Raise one arm up while lowering the other, keeping the elbows slightly bent. Alternating the arms works the anterior deltoids. 3x8 reps.

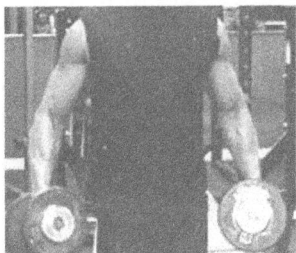

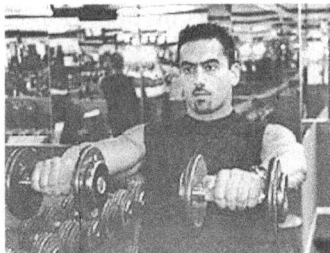

Upright Rows- Good for the traps and the anterior and lateral heads of the deltoid. Keep a straight back during this exercise. Use a shoulder- width grip, pull the bar up to your upper chest, and lower it. Do not use too heavy of a weight to keep swinging to a minimum. 3x8 reps.

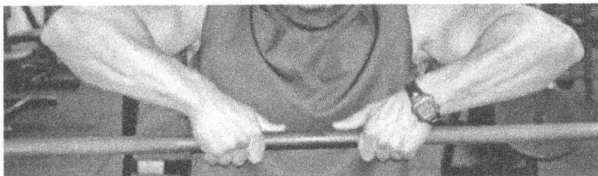

Lateral Raises – This is a great exercise for the lateral head of the deltoid. It's the only way to broaden your shoulders once you become an adult. It's excellent. Keep your arms bent at right angles, keeping your knees slightly bent, raise the dumbbell laterally to your side of the body, palms facing down. Do not use an extremely heavy weight, so you won't cheat. Don't use a jerk or momentum to raise the dumbbell. Lower to a safe level.3x8 reps.

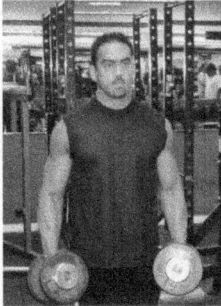

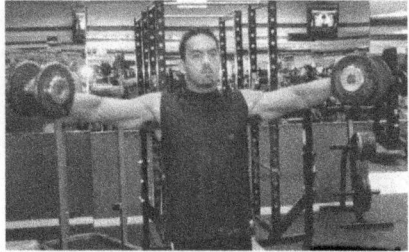

Dumbbell Press -Hold dumbbells in front of the body. Hold elbows back. Alternately press one dumbbell up as the other goes down in a continuous motion. Don't lock out at the top of movement. Good for side Deltoids. 3x8 reps.

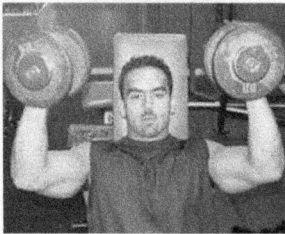

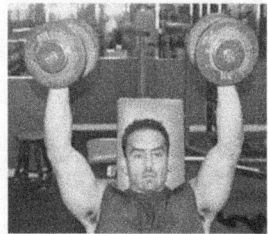

Bent over Raises- Works the rear Deltoids. Sit or bend over at the waist, grasping a pair of dumbbells. Raise your arms sideways as high as you can, without locking your elbows, making sure your palms are facing each other, and then return to starting position. 3x8 reps.

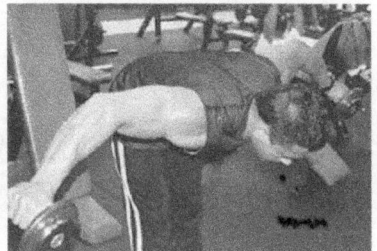

206

ARMS

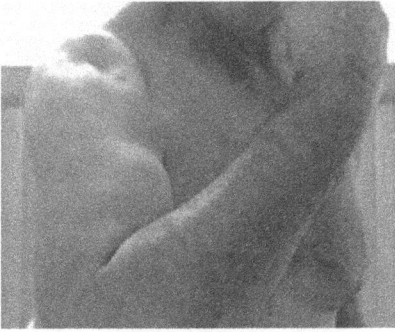

Frank Marchante arm-2023

The arms are the most exposed body part you have.

To have impressive arms, you will need to have mass, definition, and, of course, peak. When I train my arms, I like to hit biceps and triceps, supersetting one with the other.

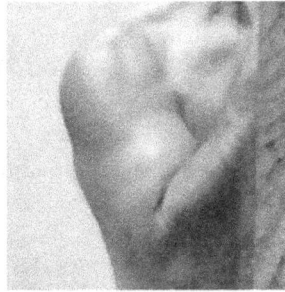

The author arm-2023

Biceps Brachii, "biceps" means "two heads"; "Brachii" means arm. One of its ends has two heads, and one is attached to your upper arm, and the other to the front of your scapula.

The biceps muscle connects two joints: the shoulders and the elbow. The biceps are used to bend your elbows and pull your forearms toward your upper arms.

The triceps brachii is a three-headed muscle that works in contrast to the biceps. It is located at the back of your upper arm. Its function is to straighten the arms. Always warm up your elbows.

Barbell Curl - The most famous of all bicep exercises and, at the same time the most productive.

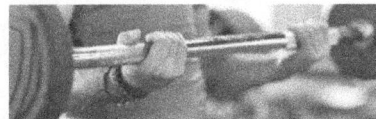

I personally like to use a very wide grip. I place my hands all the way touching the plates. Curl the bar up with your elbows close to your waist until it touches your chest. Make sure your arms are extended at the bottom to start this exercise. Lower the bar under control.3x8 reps

207

Alternating Dumbbell Curl - Sitting down on bench, curl up one dumbbell first, and then as you lower it, curl up the other hand alternating, in a continuous motion. Fantastic biceps builder.3x8 reps

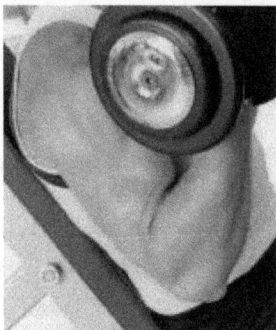

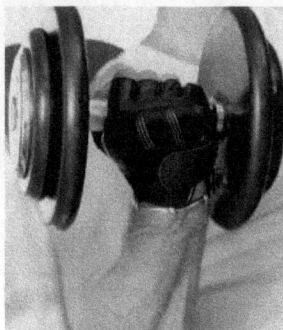

Lat High Pulldown Curl (not shown) - Sit down on a lat machine, hold the bar with medium width, and keep your elbows pointing up all the time.

Curl the bar all the way behind your neck, contract the muscle, return to the starting position and repeat. Excellent for biceps peak.3x8 reps

One-arm reverse cable pushdown (not shown): Facing the lat machine with elbow against your body, grasp the handle with palm facing up, extend or bring the arm back all the way down until it's almost completely locked out, then hold position. 3x8 reps

Lying Triceps Extensions (not shown): On a flat bench with a barbell on front of your forehead at arm's length, head held off the edge of the bench, let the bar down slowly bellow your head, pause, and return the bar up with no jerking movement to the starting position. Be careful with heavy weights and your elbows here. It is excellent for adding bulk to the upper arm. 3x8 reps.

Pulley Triceps Pushdown: Grasp a bar with hands at shoulder width. Bend your knees slightly, holding your elbows close to your body, press down, let the weight bring your arms back to the top, and repeat. You are pushing down instead of up, which means much less aggravation for your elbows. Keep this in mind if you happen to have a sensitive elbow. 3x8 reps.

Bent Over Triceps Kick back
Grasp a dumbbell with one hand and bend over at waist. Keeping the upper arm perpendicular to the floor, raise and lower the dumbbell in a continuous motion.

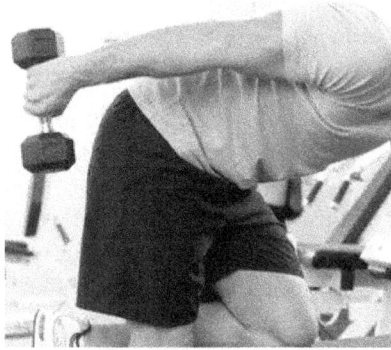

Keep upper body arm against your side or abdomen.
3x8 reps

Concentrate seated curls- holding a dumbbell and your right hand resting inside your right thigh, from this position curl the dumbbell slowly up toward your left shoulder.

At the top, contract your bicep, and pause for a few seconds, lower the weight under control to the starting position. Repeat with the other hand.
3x8 reps

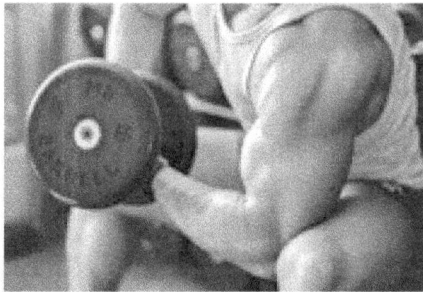

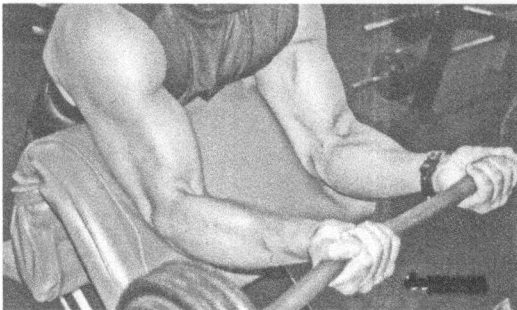

Preacher Curl-
Position your upper arms and chest against the preacher bench pad and use the biceps to curl the weight up until your biceps are fully contracted and the bar is at shoulder height. Squeeze the biceps hard and hold this position for a second. Slowly lower the bar until your upper arm is extended and the biceps is fully stretched.
3x8 reps

Forearms:

Forearms are a complex structure that can supinate, pronate, grip, extend, bend the fingers, and bend the hands into four positions. The flexor muscles are on the inside of the forearms, and the extensor muscles are on the outside or back of the forearms. Flexors are muscles that keep one body part connected to the other, and extensors are used to move a body apart, away from the other.

You will develop your forearm from your regular workout by lifting and moving weights, dumbbells, and barbells. Some champions always claimed that they got great forearm development just by training other body parts.

Forearms exercises:

Reverse curls:

Hold a barbell at about shoulder width in a similar way to a barbell curl. Only with the knuckles up. Elbows close to your side, curl the barbell up, lower it and repeat. 3x8 reps.

Wrist curl:

Sitting on a bench with your elbows resting on your legs, grab a barbell with your palm up, allow the bar to roll into your fingers, roll the bar back into your hands, move the wrist up until the forearm is contracted, lower, and repeat. 3x8 reps.

Hammer curl:

Curl dumbbell with a thump up, curl weight close to shoulder, return to starting position slowly, and repeat. Excellent for forearms and biceps peaks. 3x8 reps.

Legs

The legs are the body's largest muscles. Working your legs is very hard. Built-legs are like columns that hold a building; nothing will take more from a body than having a terrific upper body and skinny legs. Have you ever seen people like that at the beach? People can either laugh at or admire you at the beach. Most people neglect working on their legs. They spend a lot of time on the visual muscles of their arms, chest, back, and shoulders. In front of your thighs, you have a muscle group called the quadriceps, or "quads". Quadri means four and ceps means heads, so this is a four-headed muscle. The hamstrings are a large muscle on the back of your thighs, and the adductors are muscles on the inside of your thighs. The knee is the longest and most complex joint in the body.

Leg extension machine: is an excellent exercise that works the muscle structure of the front thigh (quadriceps). It shapes the quads and at the same time serves as a warm up for the more heavy-loaded leg exercises.3x8 reps.

Leg Curl: Lie face down with your heels under the padding and curl the leg up until the pads touch or are close to your gluteus. Hold and bring legs down. Don't bounce the weight up. Work the hamstrings. 3x8 reps.

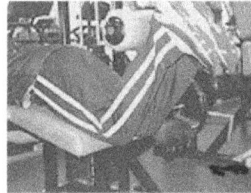

Leg press machine-Seated, press and secure your feet on the platform, unlock knees and press. Don't go to deep at bottom to protect your lower back, knees and ankles. 3x8 reps.

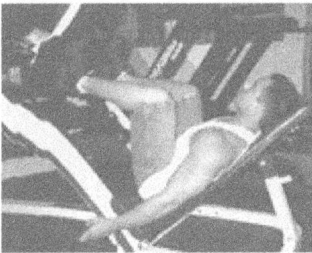
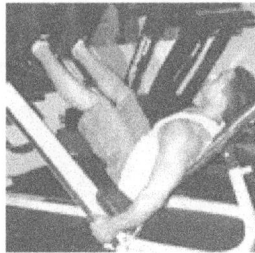

Hack Squat-Lower and raise your legs by bending and straightening your legs. Some people believe in varying the heels positions. This is an excellent exercise for the mid and lower thighs.

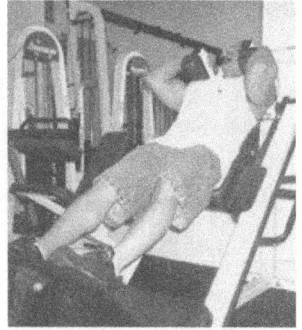

Squats

The king of exercises

The squat is a full-body muscle builder and the foremost leg and glute developer. It is very hard work, adds strength and development to the entire torso. The quadriceps (thigh muscles)work the whole body, abdominals, back, shoulders, and burn a lot of calories. You are placing a big demand on your heart, lungs and vascular system.

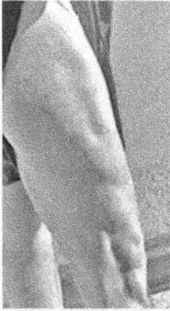

If you can do only one exercise, squats will be the one to choose. You'll get bigger, stronger, leaner. Place the bar across your back neck shoulder

Author thigh-2023 with natural feet position, shoulder-width, take a couple of deep breaths, lower yourself like you were going to sit, head straight ahead, keep your butt out, bend your knees, go down until thighs are parallel to the ground.

Exhale as you go up. Begin with a light weight to protect the joints. Be careful not to overload your knees. A slow tempo is better to avoid risk.

Squat Warning! When doing squats, do not drop down fast and do not bounce; this could damage your knees.

Calves

To develop outstanding calves, you have to do more reps than on any other body part. The lower legs must be worked constantly and progressively. You have to attack them with a vengeance, or they will refuse to grow. You must exercise the calf until you are ready to scream. You must put pressure on them and stretch them between exercises to develop a peak. It is also a good idea to walk on tiptoes every time you have a chance. The real name is gastrocnemius medial and it has two lateral heads. The soleus and the tibialis anterior are also located in the lower legs.

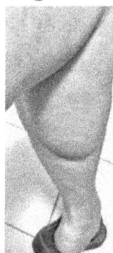

The author calf 2023

Seated Calf raises/machine: Sit on the machine with pads or barbell on your knees. Put your feet on the block, raise the toes and lower the heels to obtain a full stretch position, making sure to feel the stretch on your lower legs.

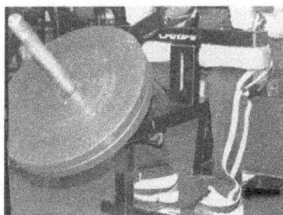

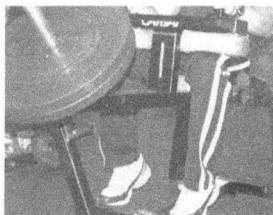

Calf raises/Machine

With barbell or machine pads on shoulders, balls of feet on block, lower heels from block and obtain a full stretch, raise as high as you can straight up with knees locked using your toes.

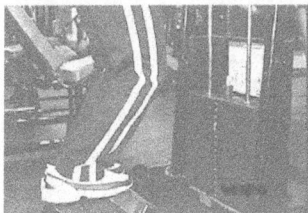

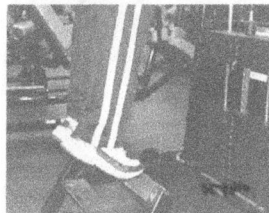

Standing Calf Rises

"To be a champion you must act like one, act like a champion"
Lou Ferrigno

Abdomen-Crunches-Vacuum

The crunch is a very basic exercise, and the great thing about it is that you don't need any equipment whatsoever. Placing your hands behind your neck, bend your legs 45 degrees, place your bottom feet flat on the floor, raise your upper body 14 degrees, exhale air, lower your body down, breathe in, and repeat without stopping.

Upper Abdominals

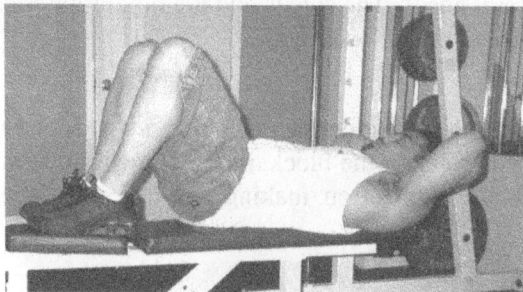

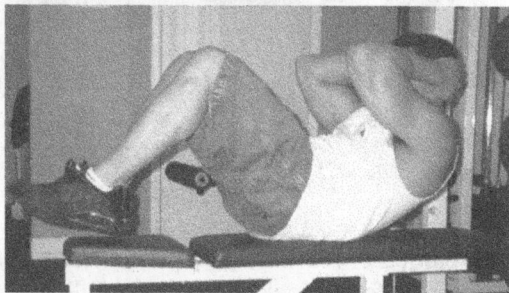

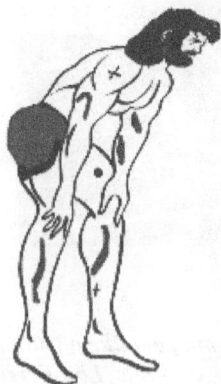

Abdominal vacuums: Bend over and place your hands on the knees or on a low bench or table, draw the abdominal muscles up into the chest cavity, let them go and relax the stomach, repeat-drawing up and relaxing, do it until you feel the stomach tire. This is a muscle control exercise that will improve your abdominal muscles 100%. Your abdominal muscles will look firmer.

Vince Gironda's favorite sit-up: Target the upper abdomen muscles.

Cross your legs in a seated position, exhale, lift your body just 1/4, tense your abdomen, do as many reps as you can, rest and repeat

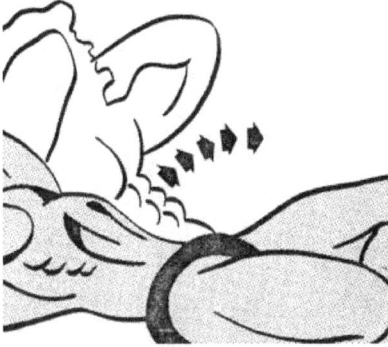

Frog sit-up

Vince Gironda's favorite: Target lower abdomen muscles.

Sit on the bench's edge, exhale. Lift your legs as high as you can, do as many reps as possible, keeping your back straight, rest and repeat.

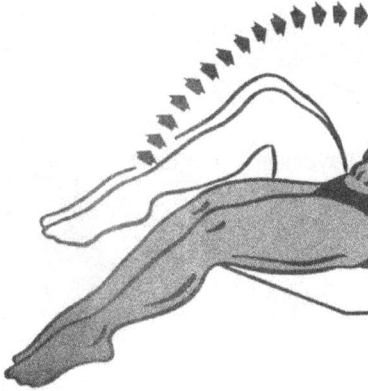

Knee pull-ins

Add ¼ to ½ inches to your arms

Many champions from the Golden Era of bodybuilding have used this method to add inches to their arms.

Dumbbell down the rack:

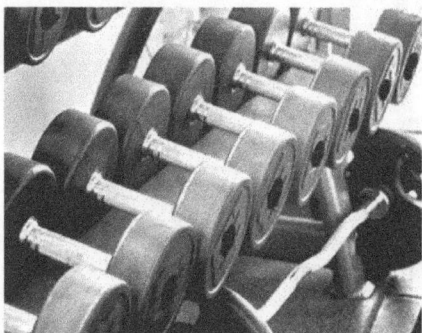

You stand in front of the dumbbell rack and pick the lightest weight and do 12 reps. Pick the next dumbbell by weight and do 10 reps. Next, pick the next one by weight and do 8 reps. Keep going down the rack to the maximum weight you can use for 1 rep. Stop to rest for a few seconds, then pick up the last dumbbell used and do 1 rep. Go back down the rack, lowering the weight and adding reps.

This is a difficult workout, so do it on one of your easier days or set aside a day just for it.

Repeat this twice a week for two or three weeks, then stop doing it for two weeks and repeat the circuit again. It worked for famous bodybuilders, and it should work for you too.

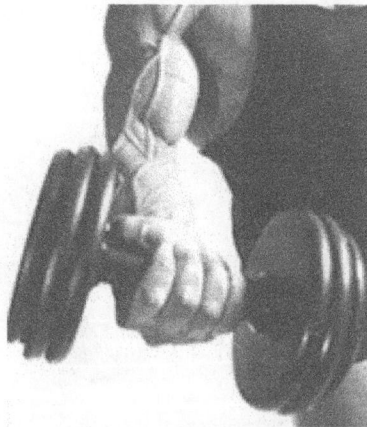

"The truest success is but the development of self"
Charles Atlas

216

Secret

Keep in mind what Sergio Oliva said in his great book, Sergio Oliva the Myth-Building the Ultimate Physique. There are no secrets. But hard workouts.

Use heavy compound exercises
Use correct repetitions

Rest-recovery time
Train cautiously

Mass training

Squat when doing Squat, do not drop down fast and do not bounce.

This could damage your knees.

Bench press: Bent-over barbell row.

Standing barbell press.

Lat machine pull down.

Barbell curl.

Routines should be changed frequently.

Change exercise often, so your body never adjusts.

You must increase resistance to add size. Period!

The Pyramid system

This is the system the great legend Sergio Oliva used. He also did

antagonist muscles like working biceps and triceps.

Injury:
It is no secret that when we grow older, it takes more time to recover, and it is easier to get hurt or develop an injury.

Focus on safety.

Concentrate when working out.
Always warm up and cool down.

Never sit down after working out or doing exercise. Walk a little bit around if you need to get your breath back.

If something hurts, stop right away and do something else. Skip that exercise for a couple of days.

If doing weight training, your first set should always be a light set.

Don't use too much weight.

Be careful

I'm going to repeat Sergio Oliva's incident here. It is much better to train with a partner than alone. Sergio Oliva tells a story in his book, Sergio Oliva the Myth- Building the Ultimate Physique, about how one time he was doing an extremely heavy bench press and he got stuck under the weight with no one around to help him. He had to roll the weight off of his body. Very scary!

Don't rush a comeback; take your time.

Remember, an injury could take months to heal and you might have to stop training for months.

Dress

You must keep your muscles warm, especially if it is cool outside. A t-shirt and shorts are OK if it is summer or warm outside. If it is cold, wear a sweet shirt, a cap, or a hat. It is very important to keep warm on winter days.

If you like an exercise, chances are you're doing it wrong.
Arthur Jones

Muscle Mass

By age 30, your muscles gradually begin to decline, especially if you don't do cardio workouts or lift weights.

The College of American Sports Medicine claims that muscle mass diminishes by nearly half during adult life. Indeed, between the ages of 50 and 70, the average woman or man loses 30% of their strength due to muscle mass loss.

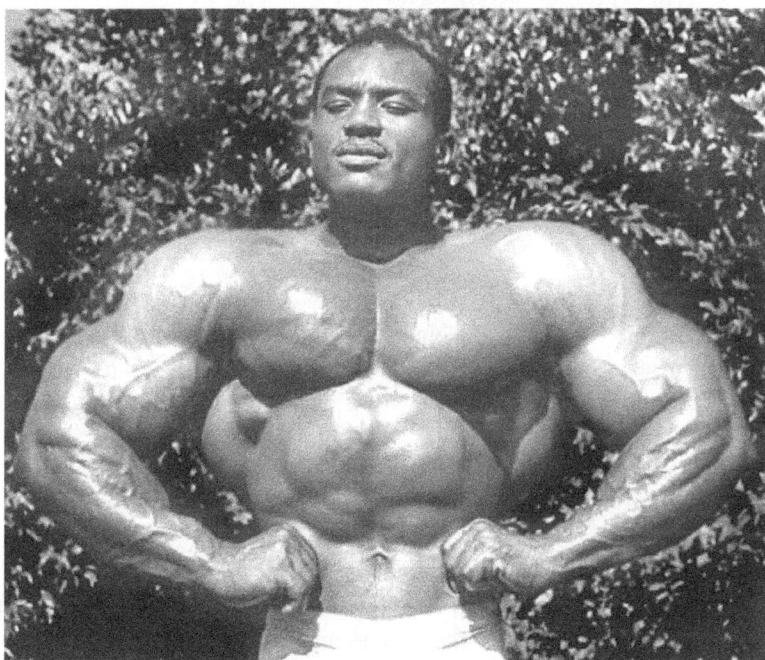

Courtesy of Sergio Oliva the Myth book-Denie photo

Even if you are inactive, muscle mass burns more calories than fat

Maintain your health and youth as long as possible!

Bulking/Mass

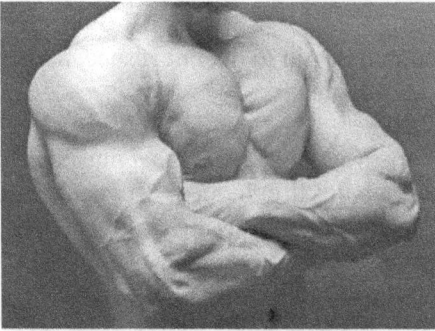

The term "bulking" is used by bodybuilders and in the fitness industry, and it means increasing your calorie intake to gain weight. Building muscle mass helps you lose weight and keep it off, and burns more calories even if you are resting. Your muscles start to deteriorate after the age of 30, especially if you don't exercise.

The American College of Sports Medicine reports that muscle mass is going to decrease by nearly half during your adult life. Don't let the statistics scare you; you can have a strong, toned, and sexy body.

Here's how:
Eat wisely
If you're trying to lose weight, remember that extreme diets produce quick results by reducing muscle mass. Slow and steady weight loss of 1 to 2 pounds each week will preserve your muscles.

Working out
Weight training combined with cardiovascular exercise quickly boosts muscle mass. The U.S. Surgeon General advocates adequate activity, such as 30 minutes of walking or 15 to 20 minutes of jogging, at least five days a week for general health. To build and preserve muscle mass, the American College of Sports Medicine recommends doing strength exercises such as weight training at least twice a week.

Consumption is what is prudent
Diets produce rapid results by reducing muscle mass, and it is almost impossible to keep that weight off. Weight loss should be gradual and consistent. Averaging 1 to 2 pounds per week is an excellent way to lose weight. Be careful what you eat. Eat with quality in mind, not quantity.

Working out/cardio

Combining weight training with cardiovascular exercises is the way to go. Even 15 to 20 minutes of jogging or fast walking at least 3 days a week is good for overall health.To build and maintain muscle mass, nothing is better than strength workouts such as weight training at least twice a week.

Compound exercises:
Lifts that work muscle at more than one joint are known as "compound exercises." These include the deadlift, squat, press, row, and pullups. Compound lifts recruit lots of muscle mass, making for efficient training and a large release of hormones such as testosterone that promote growth—make them the basics of your workouts.

There's nothing wrong with mixing in some isolation work (curls, leg extensions), but your main training should be compound lifts.
Hit all the angles of a muscle.

Pay attention to your legs:

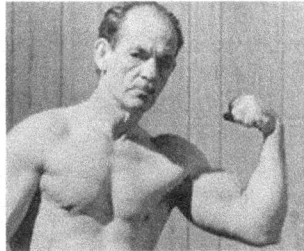

Arthur Jones

Most people new to training don't work the legs because it is much harder to workout and because they want big arms and a big chest to show now or tomorrow. Firstly, muscle imbalances look bad, and secondly, heavy compound lower-body exercises like the deadlift have an enormous impact on your overall muscular development, even in your upper body. That's because they recruit muscles everywhere, even in your shoulders and back, and they promote the release of hormones that build size and strength.

Keep in mind that you will look funny and odd in a swimming suit later, and both men and women will make comments about your skinny legs. Don't fall into this. Even if your goal is just to have a big chest and arms, you can't forget about training your legs.

I'm a hard gainer. I love weight training and have been doing it since 1962, and I had to discover the best way to train the hard way.

Stop smoking if you do, and sleep at least 8 hours every day. Don't forget to drink lots of water, close to a gallon a day.

Never use long workouts; instead, use short, hard, heavy workouts; eat a well-balanced diet; and get enough sleep. Train smart-Rest-keep an eye on warning pain

For legs
The deadlift is not a back lift as most people believe it is-look straight ahead, your spine in a flat position, not stooped or rounded. Don't try to jerk the weight.
Warm up
1-light set
1 medium set
1 heavy set
Exercises like the bent over barbell and the T-bar can be very dangerous for your low back if you jerk the weight or you are careless.

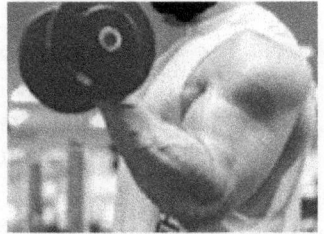
Dumbbell Curls

Best exercises:
Chins
Dips
Bent-over barbell row
Lat Pulley to the front
T-bar row
Bench Press (better inclined)
Deadlift
Dumbbell Row
Front Press
Seated Dumbbell Curls
Lateral Raises
Triceps pull down
Standing Dumbbell curls

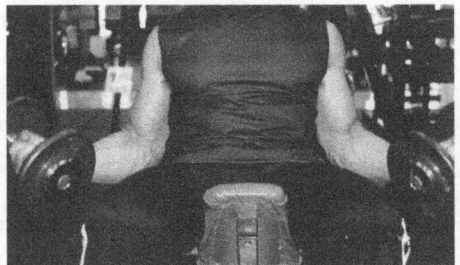
Seated Dumbbell Curls

Back

I like the one-arm dumbbell row because it protects your lower back. Place your hand on a bench or low table to relieve pressure on your lower back.

If your gym does not have a T-bar machine, just do what I do. Take a barbell and load the plates to one side, then stick the other corner of the barbell into a corner.

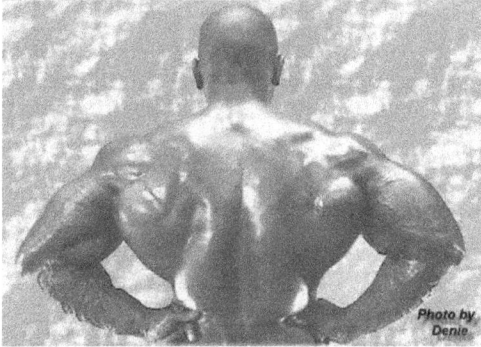

Keep your hand close to the plates and do one set with your right hand touching the plates, and then do another set with your left hand touching the plates.

Sergio Oliva back by Denie

Don't be carried away with using monstrous weights at the expense of good form and proper muscle isolation.

An improper posture is ugly and will affect your breathing and the internal organs' function. Numerous people store rolls of fat in their lower backs. Make sure to balance your back workout with your chest for balance.

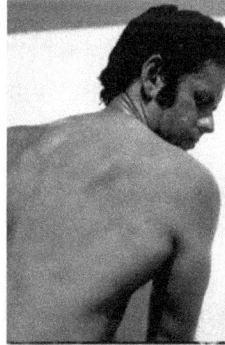

Author younger year back

"The only time we fail is when we stop trying".
Chuck Norris

MASS TRAINING

This program will make you gain at least 25 pounds of pure muscle in 4 to 5 months.
Guarantee!!!!!!!

Squat
Bench press
Bent-over barbell row
Standing barbell press
Lat machine pull down
Focus for safety- concentrate when you exercise
Warm up and cool down always
Change exercise often so your body never adjusts
Use heavy compound exercises
Use correct repetitions
Rest-recovery time
Train cautiously
Don't use to heavy weight-be always careful.
Don't rush a comeback, take your time.

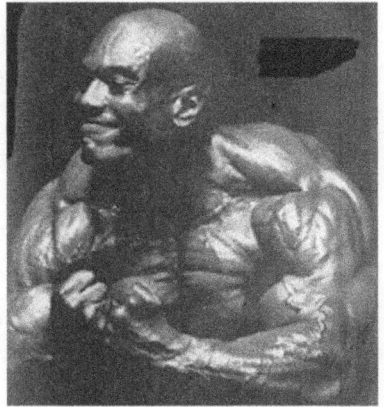

Sergio Oliva -Courtesy of Denie

Never sit down after working out or doing any exercise. Walk a little bit around if you need to get your breath back.When performing squats, do not drop down quickly or bounce; this can harm your knees.

If something hurts, stop right away and do something else. Skip that exercise for a couple of days. Try it later or discontinue it for good. When doing weights, the first set should always be a light set. Keep in mind that an injury may take months to heal and you might have to stop training for months.

Blood, sweet, and respect. The first two you give and the last one you earn.
Dwayne Johnson

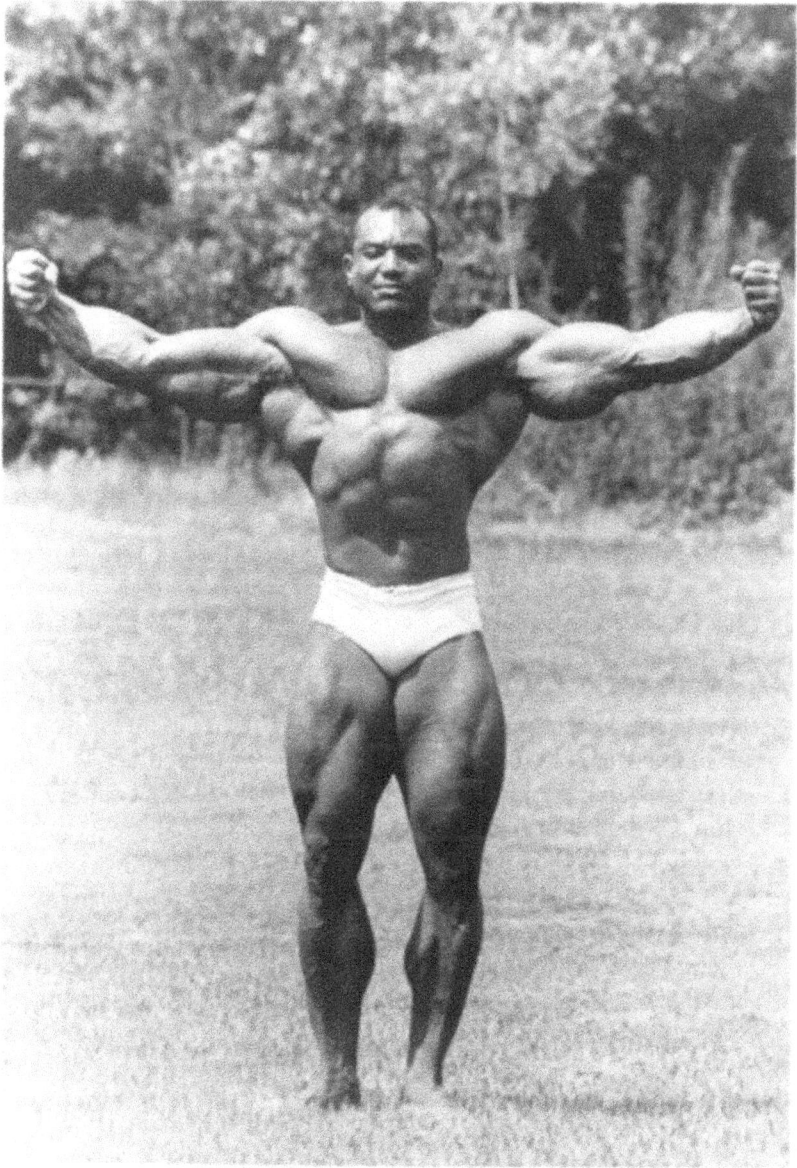

Sergio Oliva Deland Beach Fl,
Photo by Inge Cook-Jones Courtesy of Arthur Jones

Mass training

Squat Warning! When doing squats, do not drop down fast and do not bounce. This could damage your knees.

Bench press   Lat machine pull down
Bent-over barbell row   Barbell curl
Standing barbell press   Change routines often

Change exercise often, so your body never adjusts to the routine.

Pyramid system
This is the system the great legend Sergio Oliva used. He did antagonist muscles, like working biceps and triceps.

Safety concerns
Barbell Rowing
When doing the barbell rows, it is important to keep a flat lower back. Use a wide grip and pull the bar to the lower chest every now and then.

Don't use too much thrust. Be careful with heavy weights. A little thrust may possibly be okay. If you use a lot of hip thrust, you're going to use more weight, but your low back is involved with the hip thrust, placing a lot of strain on the low back. Pull the bar into your stomach. The best thing to do while doing a barbell row is use a weight you can handle.

Start each set with the bar resting on the ground, and emphasize arching your upper back. With this exercise, you have to bend a little at your knees. This exercise places your lumbar spine in a vulnerable position. Don't jerk the weight off the ground, just pull the bar up and accelerate. It will help to warm up well before you begin your barbell row.

The underhand grip for the bent-over barbell row will work less on the middle and upper back. Rows for upper back work should be done overhand with a wider grip and elbows out slightly.

Injury

It is common knowledge that as you get older, it takes longer to recover, making it easier to get hurt or develop an injury.

Concentrate on safety.

When working out, pay attention.
Always warm up and cool down.
Never sit down after working out or doing exercise. Walk a little bit around if you need to get your breath back.

If something hurts, stop right away and do something else. Skip that exercise for a couple of days.

If you are doing weight training, your first set should always be a light set.
Don't use too much weight.
Be careful.

It is better to train with a partner than alone. Sergio Oliva tells a story in his book, Sergio Oliva the Myth, Building the Ultimate Physique, about how one time he was doing an extremely heavy bench press and he got stuck under the weight with no one around to help him. He had to roll the weight off of his body. Very scary!

Don't rush a comeback; take your time. Keep in mind that an injury may possibly take months to heal, and possibly you will have to stop training for months.

Drink water during your workouts. Drink before and after exercising. Eat three good meals a day. If you can handle it, eat 6 meals a day if you are trying to gain weight.

Don't miss a workout unless you are sick.
Get sufficient rest and sleep at least eight hours every night.

What to Wear

It is necessary to keep your muscles warm, especially if it is cool outside. A T-shirt, shorts if it is summer or warm outside. If it is cold, wear a sweet shirt, a cap, or a hat. It is very important to keep warm on winter days.

Some researchers suggest the following nutrient breakdown:

Protein content ranges from 25-30%.

Fat percentage: 15-20%

55-60% carbohydrate content

Keep in mind that this is an example guide—you have to take into consideration your age, weight, height, and goals.

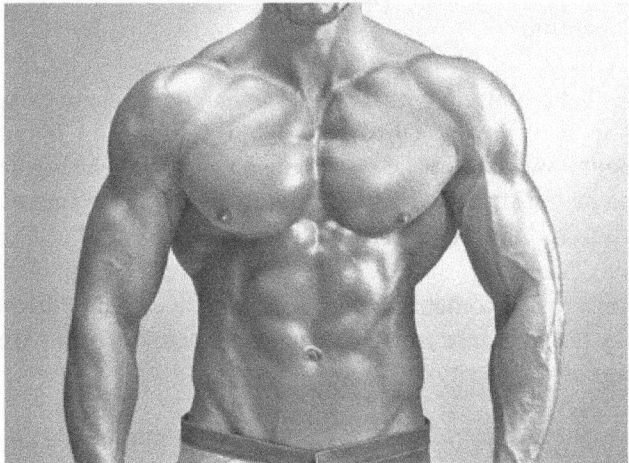

"Nobody picks on a strong man".
Charles Atlas

Old School Training to gain a massive 25 pounds of muscle

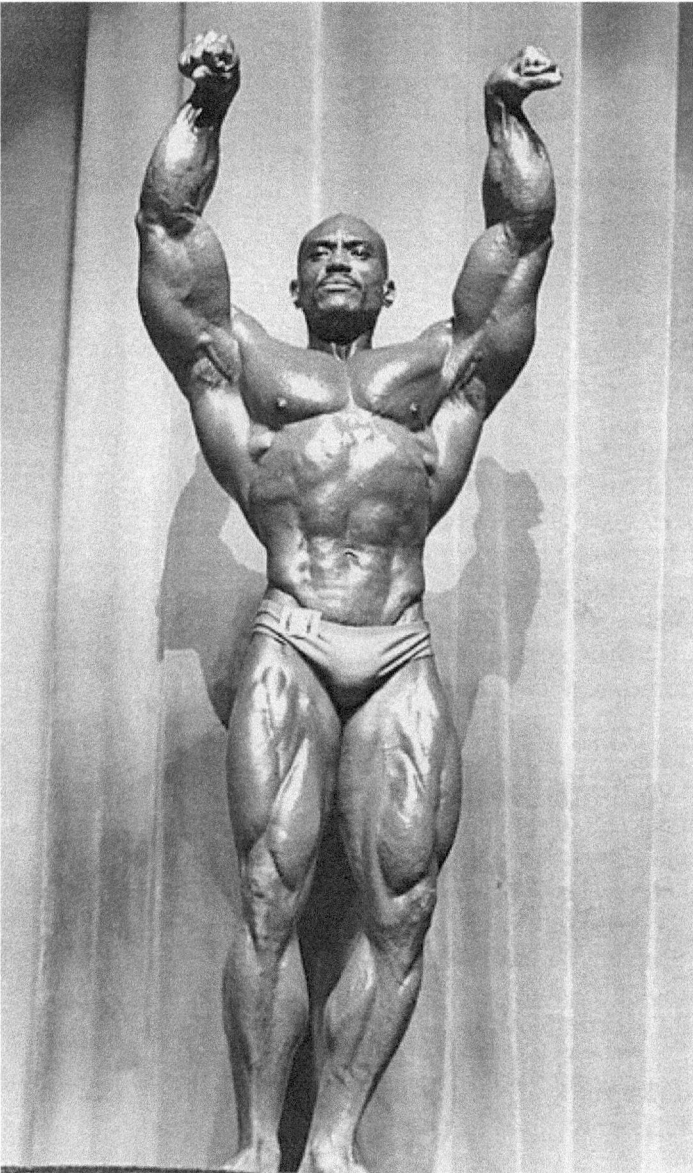

Photo courtesy Sergio Oliva the Myth book

Old-fashioned high-intensity training for men to get colossal, a huge 25 pounds of muscle.

The particular value of this **old school** training is the possibility of being able to pack on muscle mass and intensify strength more than you ever believed to be achievable. Formidable testosterone anabolic training is here.

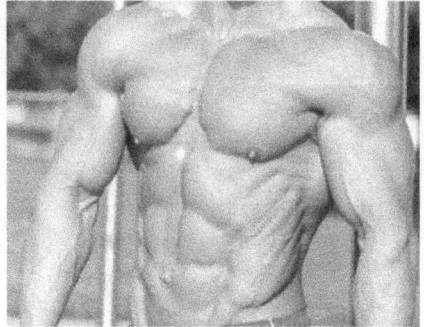

Phase #1 (week 1)
Chest
Incline press
6x5x2 – **rest** move to

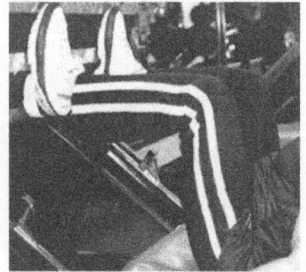

Delts
Standing Barbell Front press, Machine Press or Barbell Clean and Press (never lock elbows)
 6x5x2 **rest** move to

Lats
Palms–up pull downs
6x5x2 **rest** move to

Legs
Leg press (do not lock your knees) place your feet lower on the platform.
6x5x2 **rest** move to

Biceps
Standing Barbell curls close grip-- shoulder width grip- (**never the e z bar**)
6x5x2 **rest** move to

Triceps
Press downs bar- or rope
6x5x2

Phase #2 (week two)

Pecs-Chest
Dips toes pointing to the front, pre-exhaust –**as many as you can**
immediately go to incline press (slight bend in elbows in top
position).
6x5x2 **rest** move to

Delts
Front presses, Machine Press or Barbell Clean and Press 8x5x2(never
lock elbows) immediately go to Dumbbell lateral raises
6x5x2 **rest** move to

Lats
Palms –up pull downs 6x5x2 immediately
go to T-bar rows or Barbell Rowing palms
up 6x5x2 **rest** move to

Thighs
Leg extension for warm up 6x5x2 (do not
lock your knees) -pre-exhaust –immediately
go to Leg presses 6x5x2 –press slowly-(do
not lock your knees)-place your feet lower
on the platform **rest** move to

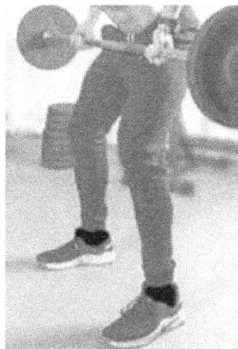
Barbell Rowing

Triceps
Press downs bar- or rope 6x5x2 pre-exhaust –immediately go to
Dips- cross legs behind as many as you can or Dip machine **rest**
move to

Biceps
Standing Barbell curls close grip
(shoulder width grip) 6x5x2
never the **e z bar** immediately go
to Dumbbell Curls 6x5x2

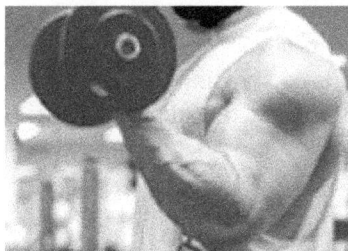
Dumbbell Curls

231

Phase 3 (week three)

Chest
Pec deck pre-exhaust —8x5x2 immediately goes to
Incline presses Bench Press-(slight bend in elbows in top position
6x5x2 **rest**

Lats
Straight arm lat pull downs 6x5x2 pre-exhaust –immediately go to
One arm dumbbell rows 6x5x2 **rest**

Shoulders
Dumbbell Press 6x5x2 (never lock elbows) pre-exhaust –immediately
go to Barbell Upright rows 6x5x2 (only to middle chest) **rest.**

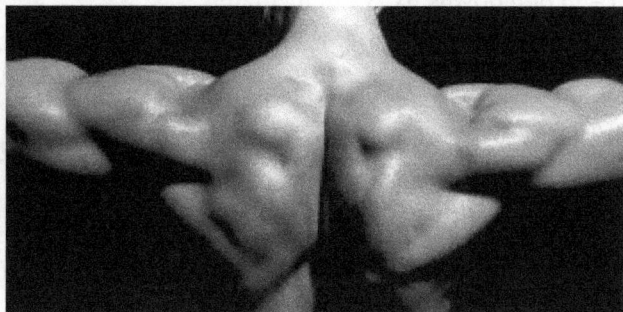

Strong muscular back

Legs
Leg extension for warm up (do not lock your knees) 6x5x2 pre-
exhaust –immediately go to
Hack Squat machine feet in the middle of the platform. (do not lock
your knees)6x5x2 **rest**

Triceps
Rope standing overhead cable triceps extension, seating or lying
triceps extensions 6x5x2 pre-exhaust immediately go to
Dips- cross legs behind as many as you can or Dip machine **rest**

Biceps
Palms –up pull downs 6x5x2 pre-exhaust –immediately go to
Barbell Cur 8x5x2

Phase 3(week three)

Whole body 3x times a week any exercise with **low** weight **high** reps.

8 reps= medium-heavy weight -but you can do about 6 more reps if you have to

5 reps= **heavy** weight - but you can do about 3 more reps if you have to

2 reps= **heavy** weight -but (**maybe**) you can do one more rep if you have to

If you finish the workout and feel like **doing more,** you are not doing a **hard workout**. Increase the **intensity**, the **weigh**t, or the **time spend doing it**. You either work hard or work long, but you can't work hard and work long. Keep your workouts brief.

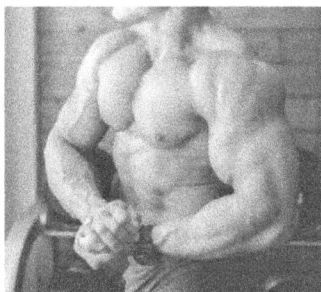

Allow maximum recuperation workouts for the **whole body** three times a week for four weeks. Repeat this routine for 8 weeks, then rearrange the exercises and start all over again for 8 more weeks.

Keep in mind that when you're working out, you're not actually building muscles, you're tearing them down. During the period of rest, your body actually builds muscles, repairing the damaged tissue.

After that, change the exercises, reps, and time and start all over from the beginning. Until you are satisfied with your new, incredible muscle mass,

Warm-up: Warm up each muscle group before blasting it. Save energy for the heavy sets—don't overdo it.

Cool down by walking around, moving your arms, and stretching only after your workout, never before, and never before you sit down.

Keep the workout as fast as possible without sacrificing rep performance. The real objective is to rest for the smallest amount of time required to recuperate for the next set, between 10 and 50 seconds on lighter sets, and 60 seconds to 120 seconds on heavier sets.

Sometimes you may rest for up to two minutes if you are doing very heavy sets, but this is not the normal majority of the time. If you are doing very heavy sets to gain bulk, you can rest a few more seconds.

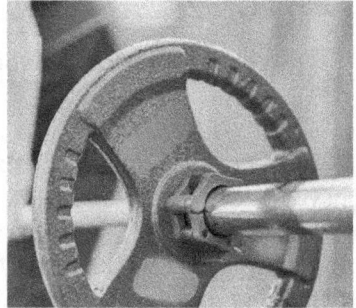

Don't use a clock during rest periods, just go by what you feel you need. Do not sit down, take a few steps, walk around, breathing until you can breathe more normally again, and then go back to your next set. Use your need for air as your guide.

The muscles get used to the same exercises and reps; we need to change the weight, reps, and sets. When you begin working out, everything works for a while. As you progress, you need more training intensity. For a new comer, it gets confusing with so many different kinds of training, like overtraining, undertraining, periodization, aerobics, volume, heavier weight, supersets, Pilates. Wahoo!for a beginner, must be really confusing.

Nothing is new or changed. The solution is hard work. Routines haven't changed, nor have the exercises, sets, and reps. Just hard, constant exercise. Never go by a clock or count the time during rest periods. Take a few steps, walk around breathing as soon as you can go back to your next set. Make your breathing or the need for air your guide.

This program will make you gain at least 25 pounds of pure muscle in 4 to 5 months, **guarantee.**

Tomorrow will be too late, it's now or never.
Elvis Presley

Eating for huge massive bulk

Grill-any meat

Top Sirloin: ranks first in terms of muscle building mass, strength, high testosterone levels, Glutamine and Creatine. **Not limit**

Bison meat is packed with protein to increase muscle mass and strength. **Not limit**

Whole eggs
Full of protein, one of the best forms of protein, each contains about 8 grams of protein (two or three a day) for larger gains in size and strength. It is **proven** that eggs does not **raise cholesterol** in young actives athletes. Over easy, poached-scrambled -boiled. **Not limit**

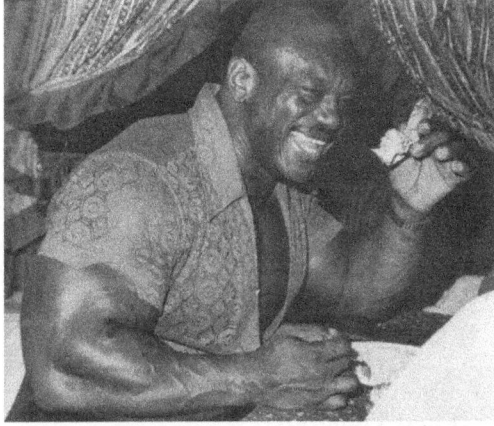

Sergio Oliva the Myth-courtesy of R. Kennedy

Chicken breast is a fat-free protein dream. **Not limit**

Fish: lean and high in protein (for mass and strength).
Tilapia-
Trout
Red Snapper

Black beans (not canned) are rich in protein, fiber, and slow digestion. Carbs enhance muscle mass. Not limit

Whole grain rice: one cup of rice with one cup of black beans contains about the same protein as a 2.5-ounce steak. One cup.

Sweet potatoes help to keep insulin stable and provide energy. One or two per day, early in the day

Backed potato fast digesting carbs- Since you are bulking up two days a week eat anything you want.

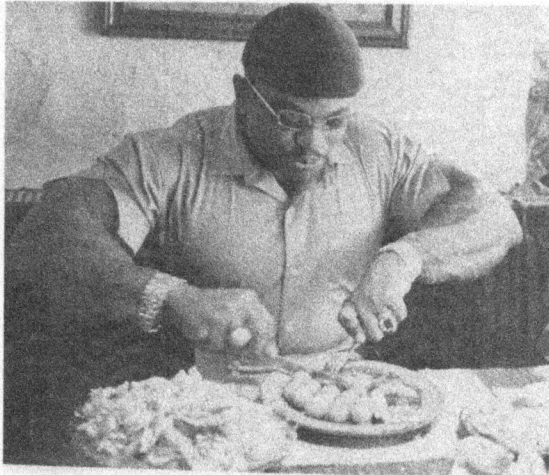

Sergio Oliva- Mr. Olympia- Mr. Universe- Mr. Olympus- Mr. America

Final Thoughts:

Eat well.

Stick with a basic, simple routine--three times a week, whole body

Heavy Weights must be lifted.

Get Rid of those Damned Abs and Eat!

If you want muscle, you need to eat a lot. If you want to be a 220lb mass monster, start eating like you weigh 220 pounds.

Learn to Stop -The most overlooked aspects of muscle building is a four-letter word: Stop

Stay warm! Get big or get out. This is old school advice. If your body is trying to get bigger, I insist you be careful about shivering, freezing, and shaking. The body is going to shift resources to produce heat.

Day snacks-beef sticks-buffalo stick-chicken sticks. **Not limit**

Greek yogurt: no flavor, contains- 18 grams of protein, three times the amount in regular yogurts- **one or two a day.**

Ice cream: ½ pint a day any flavor
Water 8 glasses a day or not limit at all.

Any fruit twice a day never in the evening or with dinner – first thing in the morning-1 hour or ½ hour before workout.

Bananas are **better**	Blueberries.
Apples	Strawberries

Juices: Orange juice-early in the day- **one cup.**
Cranberry (low sugar) to keep the **kidneys** and the **urinary** track system clean, early on the day-**one glass a day.**

Milk–one/two cups a day- **Chew** your milk instead of drinking it.

Whole bread-one/two slice

Eat slowly, always

Supplements
Vitamin E 400 mg ((dry is better) one a day

B-12 one dropper a day-or one shot a week to protect against stress and aid metabolism.

Omega-3 fatty acids one or two soft gels a day.

Argentinian Desiccated Liver vacuum dry excellent protein supplement for size and mass.4 a day.

Complete Amino Acids-one or twice a day between meals- (any)
3 days on / two days off supplements

To clean any toxics from the liver, kidneys, and stomach and to help the body use the supplement, stop using them for a few days so your body do not get used to them. Since you are bulking up, two days a week you can eat anything you want.

Fiver/Foods for Weight Loss

A-Apples

Apples slow digestion and create a full feeling longer; it's called pectin, reported nutritionists at Tufts University.

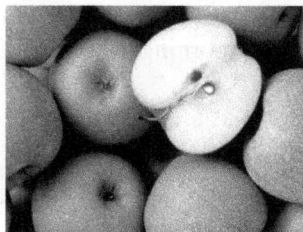

According to nutritionists at Tufts University, pectin in a whole apple is more filling than the equivalent amount of fruit in juice.

B-Eggs

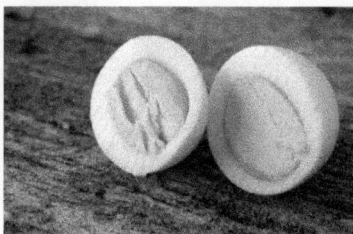

Research from Saint Louis University confirms that people who consume eggs for breakfast eat 330 fewer calories daily compared to those who have cereal, toast, or bagels for breakfast. Scholars call eggs the "complete protein," affirming that nine essential amino acids are contained within a single egg. If you have Type 2 diabetes, you must ask your doctor because research has found out that for diabetics, eggs may increase cardiovascular risk

The Academy of Nutrition and Dietetics confirms that these are the amino acids that tell your brain and body that you've attained food capacity.

C-Oats

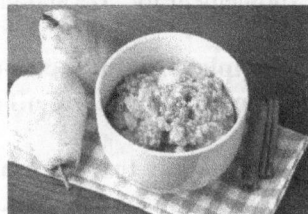

Full of high fiber; keep you satisfied for much longer.

D-Potatoes

Potatoes are starchy. However, a healthy boiled, baked, or grilled potato (not fried) will satisfy hunger. Don't overlook a grilled, baked, or boiled potato on your plate.

A potato has many nutrients like fiber, and vitamin B6, potassium, copper, vitamin C. manganese, niacin, and phosphorus.

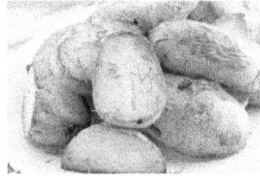

E-Greek Yogurt

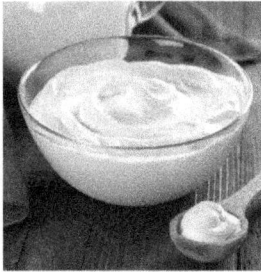

Harvard researchers published that Greek yogurt is "the sole finest food for shedding pounds." Greek yogurt balances blood sugar, curbs cravings, and keeps hungry bellies at bay for a longer period of time.

The investigation discovered that individuals that ingest Greek yogurt get rid of extra pounds without modifying their lifestyles, diets, or exercise. Remember that Greek yogurt contains double the protein and contains no whey.

F-Wheat Berries

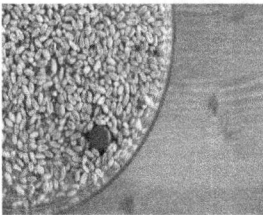

Wheat berries are full of protein and fiber. A serving contains roughly 6 grams of protein and 6 grams of fiber. Foods like wheat berries activate the release of ghrelin, a hormone that communicates to the brain that we're full.

G- Beans

Beans are good for your heart and
ideal for shaping your waistline.
Beans will fill you up. The logic is
that they absorb water during the
cooking process. They are high in
fiber and tell the brain that you're
full.

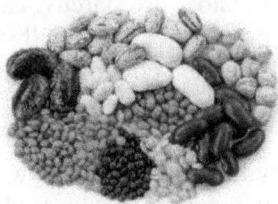

H- Lemons

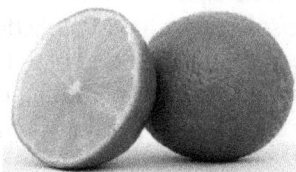

Lemons will improve the pH balance in
the intestines. Many people believe that
drinking lemon water will help them
lose weight. Findings disclose that
lemon water will improve digestion,
bowel activities, lessens appetites, and
has a sliming affect.

Although drinking lemon water as a weight loss aid has not been
proved, several studies show that improved digestion often improves
bowel movements, lessens hunger cravings, and has an overall
sliming effect.

I-Pears

Pears are packed with fiber, with roughly 6 grams
per fruit, according to a study from Washington
State University. The same Washington State
study claims pears improve healthy gut bacteria in
the colon, inhibiting Type II diabetes and
cardiovascular sickness because they're packed
with non-digestible dietary fiber, which aids
the stability of normal metabolic processes.

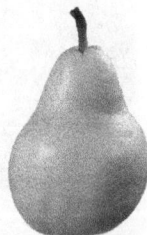

J- Avocado

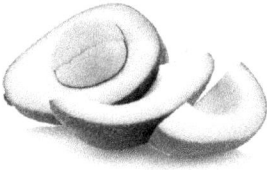

The report of the Nutrition Journal reveals that avocados contain beneficial plant-based fats that enhance cardiovascular health, are rich in fiber, fill you up, reduce inflammation in the body, and lower the pain of arthritis.

K-Broth-Based Soups

Both chicken rice soup and lentil soup are broth-based. Both are high in water content and rich in fiber. The European Journal of Clinical Nutrition reports that pureed or blended broth-based soups keep you full longer because they digest more slowly than solid meals and chunkier soups.

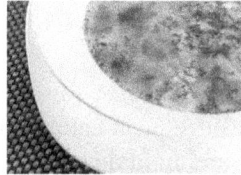

K- Fish

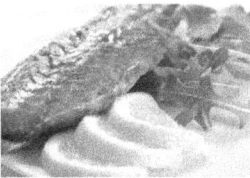

Fish provide lean protein. Fish are packed with lean protein, healthy omega-3 fats, and amino acids.

L- Beef

Lean beef is high in protein. Consuming lean cuts of red meat in moderation is permissible. However, the high saturated fat content should be avoided. The best lean cuts are tenderloin, top round, and sirloin.

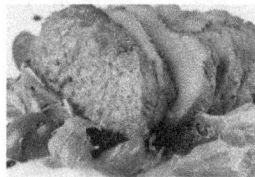

M- Leeks

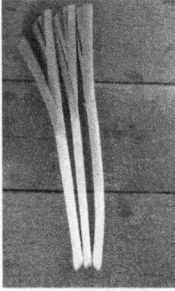

The data from the American Gut Project (AGP) shows that lightly steamed, sautéed, or raw leeks have tons of benefits, both mentally and physically. The dietary fiber in leeks will boost healthy bacteria in the colon and aid digestion.

Rules for Nutrition

1) Eat every few hours.
Infrequent eating makes your body kick into a panic-survival mode and hold on to the weight. Instead, eat smaller meals every 2.5 to 3 hours.

2) Consume fiber.
Eating foods with plenty of fiber keeps your blood sugar at a consistent level, so you crave fewer junk foods.
Consume healthy fats.

3) Healthy fats
Aid in fat loss, protect your muscle mass, and help with mental clarity and focus, vitality, and longevity.

4) Calories
Do not over-eat when you are trying to lose weight.

5) Don't deprive yourself!
Use common sense and moderation to have a favorite cheat food once or twice a week. Your results will come quicker if you enjoy the process without completely depriving yourself.

"A healthy outside starts from the inside".
Robert Urich

Ideas to Cut Calories to Avoid Gaining Weight

When cooking, make substitutions. Pick the right beverages and eat lower-calorie healthy foods.

Use low-salt.

Drink plenty of water and stay away from sodas, sweet teas, and sugary sports drinks.

Skip the sugar or use a zero-calorie sweetener instead.

Choose skim or 2% milk, wheat crackers over butter crackers, grilled chicken over crispy chicken, and yogurt over ice cream.

Portion Size- keep an eye on French fries and big sodas.

Eat salads and watch out for toppings and dressings. Use a low-fat dressing or switch to a vinaigrette.

Alcohol is another source of hidden calories. For health reasons, women should have no more than one drink a day, while men should stop at two.

Replace pasta with whole grain pasta or vegetables, such as spaghetti squash or zucchini shreds.

Yo-yo diet theory

Yo-yo is a term coined by Kelly D. Brownell at Yale University to discuss weight loss and weight gain, bringing to mind the up and down motion of a yo-yo. The individual first loses weight, then gains the weight back. The dieter tries again to lose the weight, and the cycle starts again. That's why diets don't work.

There's no need to count calories; just select **"clean"** foods.

Protein:

Lean steak
Grilled chicken breasts
Turkey breast
Baked or grilled fish
Veggies green veggies, broccoli, etc.
Starch sweet potato, whole-wheat pasta
Salad with Olive Oil and Vinegar dressing
Turkey Breast sandwich
Dessert fruit
The answer to an athletic, sexy, and strong body is portion size and quality food.

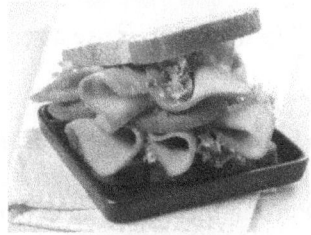

Generally, people do yo-yo dieting—a cycle of weight loss followed by fat gain, followed by more weight loss and then more fat gain. Physicians allege that it takes about 20 minutes for your stomach to "know" it's full. Now you know why you eat until you're full, and then 20 minutes later feel completely stuffed.

"One should eat to live, not live to eat"
Benjamin Franklin

On the Go

Great Tips:

Keep fresh fruit nearby. They are low in calories. Some are apples, grapes, pears, and bananas.

Try to eat natural foods.

Bring veggies, salad, or soup to work.

Being active Take walks, use the stairs or go to the gym.

Learn what to eat for a snack.

Good snacks: pretzels, popcorn.

Fiber

Fruits, vegetables, and whole grains are fiber-rich; low-fat dairy is a great choice.

Why Should You Eat Oatmeal? Oats have both soluble and insoluble fiber. The insoluble fiber in oats helps provide a "moving" ability by curtailing constipation and improving intestinal health.

One cup of cooked oatmeal contains about 150 calories, four grams of fiber (about half soluble and half insoluble), and six grams of protein. Oats deliver essential minerals. Oatmeal contains thiamin, magnesium, phosphorus, zinc, manganese, selenium, and iron.

Oats are gluten-free, but check with manufacturers to ensure that their products are gluten-free. Oatmeal can aid weight loss by keeping you feeling fuller for longer.

Sadly, carbs are frequently dreaded by people trying to drop a few pounds, but keep in mind that by choosing whole grains, you can control hunger. But it is important to consider portion sizes.

Sugar

Food companies disguise sugar in their products under different names. So here is a list of a few. Keep your eyes open.

Corn Sugar
Dextrose
Glucose
Sucrose
lactose
Maltose is a sugar replacement.
Raw Sugar
And many more.

Carbohydrates: There are two kinds of carbohydrates: simple and complex. The simple carbs found in cakes, sugar, candy, and cookies are those you must stay away from. Complex carbs are usually full of fiber, photochemicals, vitamins, and minerals. Both are beneficial.

Salt: In reality, salt is needed by everybody to function correctly. You simply need a very small quantity. The problem is the amount of salt people use today; the companies add salt to all processed food.

Fiber-Most people are not getting adequate fiber today. People on a diet low in fiber are going to get constipation, hemorrhoids, polyps, and maybe cancer of the colon.

Food-The amount of food you should be eating must be determined by your size, condition, needs, and plans. You want to add weight? You want to reduce weight? You want to gain muscle bulk? It all depends on you.

Fats-There are polyunsaturated fats and monounsaturated fats. Monounsaturated fats reduce bad cholesterol, reducing the danger of a heart attack.

Muscle burn more calories than fat

A vigorous person with muscle mass burns more calories while sitting than a sedentary person with fewer muscles.

Balance is crucial when it comes to how much fat to eat.

Good Fats

Monounsaturated fats are healthy fats that can help reduce bad cholesterol levels, reduce the risk of heart disease and decrease inflammation. Foods that are good are avocados, nuts and nut oils, olive oil, and canola oil.

Polyunsaturated fat: It lowers total cholesterol. Vegetable oils such as corn, safflower, sunflower, and soybean oil are rich in polyunsaturated fats. Fatty fish is a rich source of heart-healthy polyunsaturated fat called omega-3 fatty acids.

Bad Fats

Saturated Fat: It raises cholesterol and causes heart disease. Foods rich in saturated fats include butter, full-fat dairy products, and red meat.

Trans Fat: Trans-fat is found in partially hydrogenated oils and gives cookies, chips, and crackers a long shelf life.

The National Academy of Sciences concluded that trans fats raise blood cholesterol. Avoid them.

The Healthiest Oils: Canola, soybean, corn, sunflower, and safflower oils. These oils are rich in heart-healthy mono-or polyunsaturated fats. Focus on natural foods--whole foods like raisins, nuts, and fresh fruit.

Conclusion:

- Testosterone production is affected by diet, exercise, stress, and supplements.

- Eat a high-protein, healthy-fat diet.

- Reduce your stress, drink plenty of water, and get enough sleep.

- Consider supplements to increase the body's ability to make testosterone.

- Train with weights on your whole body for exercises that require large muscles.

- Short-duration exercise has been confirmed to enhance testosterone levels and slow its decline.

Strength Training: Strength training, as we have discussed earlier, is known to boost testosterone levels, provided you are doing it intensely.

Sugar should be limited or avoided in your diet.

Tuna-Tuna is a heart-healthy, protein-rich food that's low in calories. Either canned or fresh, eating tuna can be a natural way of boosting testosterone. Keep in mind that eating too many omega-3 fatty acids from fish and from other foods may increase your risk of prostate cancer.

Low-Fat Milk with Vitamin D: Milk is a complete supply of protein and calcium. Children and women should drink milk for better bone health. Drinking milk can help men get strong bones. It is a good idea to drink fortified milk with vitamin D. If you're trying to lose weight, this is superior to skim milk.

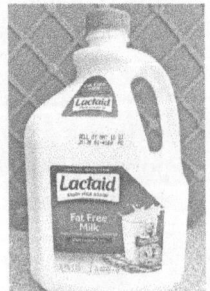

Egg Yolks: Egg yolks are a very rich source of vitamin D. A few years back, eggs gained a bad reputation because of cholesterol. Not anymore. Some experts claim that the cholesterol in egg yolks may even help with low T.

If you don't have cholesterol problems, you can eat one egg per day safely. Check with your doctor anyway. If you have Type 2 diabetes, you must ask your doctor because research has found that for diabetics, eggs may increase cardiovascular risk.

Beef: Many people have health concerns about eating red meat. Eating excessive amounts of meat is linked to cancers, such as colon cancer. Nevertheless, certain beef cuts have some nutrients that can help lower T. Beef liver is an excellent source of vitamin D, while ground beef possesses zinc.

Make sure to choose lean cuts of beef and don't eat it every day.

Beans: Black beans, white beans, kidney beans, and all are good sources of vitamin D and zinc. These foods are full of plant-based proteins that can protect heart health.

Many elderly people are deficient in vitamin D. Probably because of their age, they spend less time in the sun. Studies show the risk of vitamin D deficiency in people over 65 years of age is very high.

Surprisingly, a great number of older people who live in sunny climates don't have enough vitamin D in their bodies.

Source: Vitamin D-Mayo Clinic

Side effects of taking vitamin D may include:
Nausea and vomiting
Poor appetite and weight loss
Indigestion
Confusion and disorientation
Heart rhythm problems
Kidney stones and kidney damage.

Vitamin D can cause problems with some medications used to treat high blood pressure and heart conditions. Never take vitamin D without first asking your doctor. People with some conditions should be careful when considering taking vitamin D. Here is a list of some precautions:

High blood calcium or phosphorus levels
Heart problems
Kidney disease
Tuberculosis
Some studies claim that when you have sex more often, you help keep testosterone levels high, and when you have higher testosterone levels, you want to have sex more often, concluding that frequent ejaculation boosts testosterone levels.

Obtain plenty of sleep. Sleep helps with muscle-building hormones, particularly growth hormones and testosterone. When you sleep plenty, you have more energy, and you will have higher hormone levels. Get at least 7–8 hours of sleep per night.

Ginseng: Ginseng is a potent root that helps you with many healthful functions. The Chinese have used it for centuries to increase libido and testosterone. Ginseng promotes the central nervous system and gonadal tissues and will help with erections in males. Ginseng contains ginsenosides that boost the conversion of arginine to nitric oxide and will help build muscle mass.

You have three similar herbs called ginseng: Asian or Korean ginseng (Panax ginseng), American ginseng (Panax Quinquefolius), and Siberian "ginseng" (Eleutherococcus Senticosus).Asian ginseng is a perennial herb similar to the shape of the human body. Most people believe ginseng is a stimulant.

In traditional Chinese herbology, Panax ginseng was consumed to improve digestion, the lungs, calm the spirit, and increase overall energy. Amazingly, traditional Chinese medicine, where ginseng comes from, does not entirely agree. According to some researchers, Korean red ginseng may have some benefits for impotence and erectile dysfunction sufferers.

MENS HEALTH

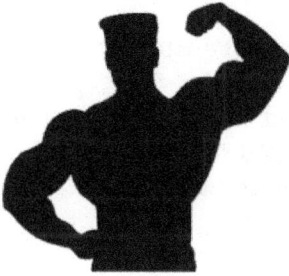

Testosterone and men
Research indicates that 60% of men over 65 have free testosterone levels below the average values of men aged 30 to 35. As a man ages, there's a slow and steady reduction in testosterone production.

A low testosterone value should be verified by a reliable test center. The inconvenience is that there is not a universal test between labs when it comes to assessing this. Several labs use one technique, but another laboratory will use a different test. When values are less than 200 or 250 ng/DL, they are considered low.

Several clinical estimates suggest the normal lower range for total T is 170 to 200 ng/dL. This is much lower than the 300 ng/DL maximum established in the past 30 years by conventional techniques. The final calculation should be concluded after various tests, not just one.

If you learn you are suffering from low T, consult your doctor and ask him/her about taking vitamin D3. New studies have confirmed that vitamins D3 and E will help to increase testosterone levels.

Omega-3s (EPA and DHA)
The omega-3 fats EPA and DHA are found in fish oil and are needed for hormone production by testosterone. Omega-3s also have anti-inflammatory effects, and you will recover quicker after training.

Summary
It is proven that testosterone production is improved by diet, exercise, and supplements.
Eat a moderately high-protein, healthy-fat diet.
Weight training
Lower your stress.
Drink plenty of water.

Make sure you get enough sleep. Study supplements to naturally produce testosterone. A short, hard workout has proved helpful in increasing testosterone levels and slowing down its decline.

An example of a typical high-intensity routine:

Warm up for three minutes – walk around, move your arms, throw some punches. Exercise as fast as you can for 20 seconds. Recover and walk for 60 seconds. Make the fast exercise and recovery longer each week until you can do 7 or 8 sets at once.

You can use any exercise like jumping jacks, or any equipment like a stationary bike, a treadmill, or even sprinting in the yard. Start slowly to avoid injury, working your way up, especially if you are out of shape.

Consume plenty of zinc supplements. Findings reveal that zinc helps with testosterone production.

Tuna is rich in vitamin D and is a protein-rich food low in calories. You can choose canned or fresh; it is up to you. A number of reports tell us that eating too many omega-3 fatty acids from fish may increase your risk of prostate cancer. Be careful.

Study supplements to naturally produce testosterone. A short, hard workout has proved helpful in increasing testosterone levels and slowing down its decline.

"One cannot actualize his goals until he visualizes them clearly in the minds eye"

Mike Mentzer

Some theories about why we age, lose ability, and die.

The genetic component

The theory of free radicals

Theory of waste accumulation

The cell-limited theory

Hayflick theory

Death by hormone theory

Mitochondrial theory

The error and repair theory

DNA theory

Autoimmune theory

Calorie restriction theory:

The gene mutation theory

The theory of living rates

A Theory of Disturbance

Telomerase theory

Cross-linkage theory

Neuroendocrine theory

Thymic Stimulating Theory

Personally, I believe the truth is probably in a mix of all these theories, but I personally believe in the Thymic Stimulating Theory.

When we are born, the dimension of this gland is about 200 to 250 grams, and when we are about 60 years old, this gland is about three grams. Some scientists believe that the reduction of the thymus could be a process of aging. Scientifics have used growth hormone to reverse thymus shrinking in mice and also have similar results with dogs. Also, they believe that if the thymus gland were to return to its regular size, the potency of youth would return in adulthood

This gland is located in the chest and produces t-cells, which are essential to fight infection and protect the autoimmune system.Check all the theories and make your own decision

Remain young: Remaining young is a state of mind. I feel very young. I believe it is because I worked 30 years with young people. I'm convinced that this kept me young, listening to new music and making new jokes. I saw new clothes, talked, and thought I was young.

AGE: Age decline is inevitable. Up-to-date training techniques and new nutritious products give you the option of maintaining youth and agility and a body in shape past your chronical age.
About 77% of Americans now alive were born after 1939. The diseases that affect most of us fall into three categories: Among the most common are inherited genetic diseases, infectious diseases, and trauma. Early detention is the key to beating the heart, cancer, and most diseases.

Baby-boomers: The baby-boomer generation, born between 1946 and 1964, chooses to stay active and keep their ability to exercise, live a healthy life, and enjoy life. This is my generation, and I'm proud to be a baby boomer.

Plan

Avoid stress as much as possible.

Exercise for 30 minutes at least every day.

Get 7 to 8 hours of sleep.

Stop smoking—don't smoke.

Drink eight or more glasses of water every day.

Limit your alcohol consumption.

Eat healthy.-Slow down your pace while eating.

Keep an eye on the portion sizes.

I have a bowel movement every day.

Avoid strong chemical smells.

Take care of your eyes and teeth.

Protect your ears

GH

When you are young, your hormones work to regulate many body functions. Once we get older, the growth hormone declines, causing us to lose muscle, body weight, and body fat.

As we age, HGH-Testosterone and the thyroid hormone will drop. There are findings that HGH declines in every animal species that has been evaluated to this date. According to the findings, by the age of thirty-one, HGH declines by about 14% per decade, and by the age of sixty-one, it is about half.
Why the decrease? Scientists and physicians still do not have this answer.

HGH regenerates the immune system. Improves sexual function in both males and females, who report improved sexual function. People look younger. HGH is not a magic bullet, because most experiments come from animals.

HGH is a drug and can only be prescribed by a doctor. Extended after-effects are unknown. The side effects are carpal tunnel syndrome, high blood pressure, growth of small breasts in men, and impotence. Additionally, the risk of spurring cancerous cell growth is present in the body. Caution is a must!!!

Natural HGH releases

Investigations have indicated that the amino acid argentine stimulates the pituitary gland to release HGH. Also, the amino acid ornithine causes the same stimulation. Many think combining both of these amino acids works better to release natural HGH.

Exercise has been demonstrated to be an excellent way to increase HGH release. High intensity bodybuilding three or four times a week will raise your HGH levels. Heavy weights rather than lighter loads seem most effective for releasing HGH. Likewise, lower body exercises are the most effective for releasing HGH. It seems like HGH response is better to strenuous activities.

DHEA (Dehydroepiandrosterone)

DHEA is produced by the adrenal gland and also declines as we age. By 60, your body is only producing about 10 to 15% of what it did in your younger years. Numerous scientists believe that restoring

DHEA's health and vigor could be restored.

Side effects are not well documented; specialists do not suggest using it if you have prostate problems, cancer, or liver damage.

Estrogen is one of the female hormones that regulate menstruation, fertility, and menopause.

Testosterone is the main hormone produced by the testicles. After puberty, testosterone drops gradually in men.

Testosterone promotes:

Promotes sexual desire.

Aggressiveness.

Stimulates growth.

It promotes protein anabolism to build muscle.

Stimulates sperm.

Bone mass

Consumption of calcium, vitamin D, and sunlight, particularly when we are young, will increase bone mass.

The main systems of the human body are:

The circulatory/cardiovascular system includes the heart, the blood, and the blood vessels.

The dermal/integumentary system includes the skin, hair, and nails.

The digestive or gastrointestinal system includes the mouth, pharynx, esophagus, stomach, liver, gall bladder, pancreas, small intestine, large intestine, the rectum, and the anus.

The Endocrine/Glandular Hormonal System includes all of the glands in the body.

Lymphatic system/Immune system-Defends the body against pathogens that may endanger the body.

The muscular system includes the muscles and tendons of the body.

The nervous system includes the brain, spinal cord, and nerves of the body.

The excretory system, which includes the renal system, urinary system, and large intestine, is the system where the kidneys filter blood.

The male reproductive system includes the testes and the penis. In a female, it includes the ovaries and the uterus.

The respiratory system includes the nose, mouth, pharynx, larynx, trachea, bronchial tubes, and the lungs.

The skeletal system includes all of the bones, joints, ligaments, and tendons of the body.

The vestibular system provides the sense of balance and spatial orientation for the purpose of coordinating movement with balance.

"The first wealth is health".
Ralph Waldo Emerson

"Where's the beef?"

A new study in 10/2020 discloses that eating beef is not as bad as believed. Lean beef is high in protein. A 4-ounce sirloin steak offers amino acids and over 30 grams of protein. Eating lean cuts of red meat in moderation is fine; just keep it on average to avoid the high saturated fat content.

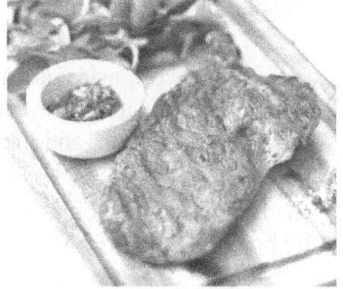

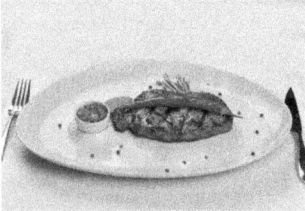

The best lean cuts are tenderloin, top round, and sirloin.

Many people have health concerns over eating red meat. Eating excessive amount of meat is linked to cancers, such as colon cancer. Nevertheless, certain beef cuts can be very nutritious Beef liver is an excellent supply of vitamin D, while ground beef possess zinc.

Make sure to choose lean cuts of beef and don't eat it every day. Many people have reservations about the consumption of red meat.

The general belief is that red meat can be bad. A recent finding from 10/2019 shows that eating three ounces a day of lean red meat was not connected with a bigger risk for heart disease or diabetes.

Small cuts of red meat are beneficial; the suggested portion size for lean red meat is three to four ounces.

Organic, grass-fed lean beef, richer in omega-3s, vitamin E, and linoleic acids, is the healthiest type of red meat to eat.

Bodybuilders eat plenty of meat to grow, and put on muscle weight. Select lean cuts of beef and avoid eating it every day.

Meat isn't as unhealthy for you as was once believed.

Small amounts of red meat are actually really good for you; it's a great source of protein and helps your body perform necessary functions (like breathing).The suggested serving size for lean red meat is three to four ounces, about the size of a deck of cards. The most beneficial type of red meat for you is organic, grass-fed lean beef, which is more abundant in omega-3s, vitamin E, and linoleic acids than conventional beef.

The Unhealthiest Type of Red Meat: One of the worst types of red meat for you is ham. This variety of red meat is high in fat (7.7 grams of fat, with 2.7 grams of saturated fat) and sodium (1.275 milligrams of sodium, which is about half of the daily recommended amount).

Nutritious Value: A three-ounce serving of red meat (beef) delivers you with half (about 25g) of your suggested daily protein intake and is also a tremendous source of vitamins B6 and B12 (which give you energy), zinc (which helps maintain your immune system), and a good supply of iron (which helps your body use oxygen efficiently).

Heart Health: Contrary to general belief, red meat does not increase the risk of coronary disease. A new study shows that eating three ounces a day of lean red meat was not linked with a higher risk of heart disease or diabetes.

Most Common Cuts: The five most popular cuts are: chuck pot roast, top loin steak (a.k.a. New York strip), top round steak, and T-bone steak.

Red Meat Varieties: We think of red meat as beef, pork, and venison, but it also includes goat, lamb, buffalo, bison, and ostrich.

Popular Variety: Beef is the most popular red meat in the U.S., but **goat meat** is the most popular red meat in the **rest of the world**.

Pork tenderloin is one of the healthiest cuts of red meat, contains about 122 calories per serving, and is rich in protein and B vitamins.

If you want to lose fat, get lean, strong and ripped, These are six mistakes to avoid.

The first mistake: isolated exercises.

Performing isolated exercises like bicep curls will not get you results. One-muscle-at-a-time simply doesn't increase your calorie burn.

Second mistake: working out with machines

Machines are great. The problem is this: machines change the way your body physically moves, controlling and restricting your motion. Some machines can cause an excessive burden on your joints.

3rd mistake--Cardio for extended periods of time

The truth is, you need to do cardio if you want to lose weight and burn fat, but you must take precautions against pounding the pavement and sore joints.

4th mistake: Sit-Ups

For years, individuals believed that doing traditional ab exercises like crunches and sit-ups would get them a six-pack. This was not true. They don't burn any fat.

5th mistake-repeated over and over

Why keep doing the same old workouts that haven't gotten any results? If you want to keep making progress in your body, you've got to start changing your workouts.

Mistake number six: Extensive Workouts-Believe me, the trick is shorter, faster, and more rigorous workouts. Too much aerobics will reduce your muscle-building development. Running is not a muscle builder and is only used at the beginning of the conditioning phase.

Glutes

Sleek, strong and sexy

Glutes are a part of your lower body strength and development. A

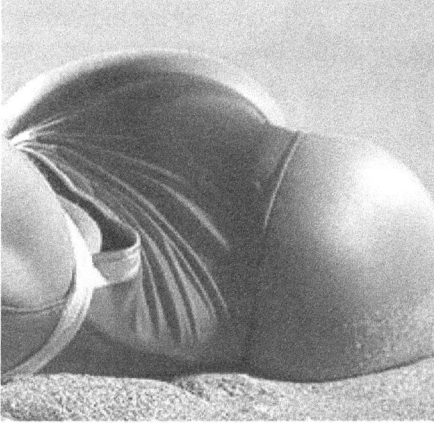

muscular posterior is also essential for symmetry and a large part of your appearance. Imagine wearing jeans, a bikini, mini-skirts, or shorts. Most people do not do any direct glue work, which is a mistake, especially for a woman. Exercises for the glutes should be included in every training routine for men and women.

Genetic Factors:

Some women have naturally larger lower bodies compared to their upper bodies, probably because of genetics. The biggest challenge to shaping the female physique is leaning out the lower body. Another genetic factor is having a tendency to store fat in the lower body by inherently having more fat cells in the hips, thighs, calves, and glutes.

If you would like to increase your leg size, you need to do high-intensity, short-duration activities.

If your legs are too big, experts believe that long distance running is the ideal action for leaning your lower body mass. If your goal is to slim your lower body down, make sure that your lower body participates in low-intensity, long-duration exercise on a regular basis.

I totally believe that long-distance running is the perfect activity for eating away your lower body mass.

Gluteus Maximus Muscle Function

The functions of the gluteus maximus are extension, lateral rotation, and adduction of the hip joint. The speedier you run, the further your gluteus maximus gets worked. This is the reason marathon runners aren't recognized for having a great ass; they don't acquire a great ass because they're not training it with enough intensity to tap into all of the muscle fibers.

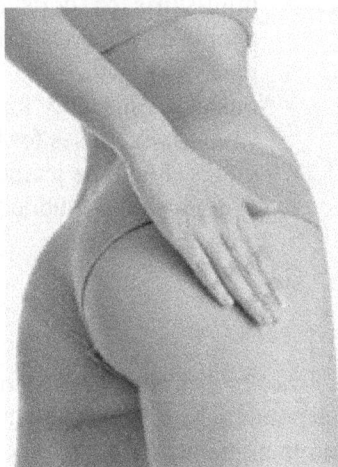

Once you walk, you plant your leg in front, the other being pulled back as you propel forward. This is what the gluteus maximus is intended to do. To run, you need to pull your leg back very quickly. The speedier you run, the more your gluteus maximus gets worked.

Remember, a sprinter does hundreds or thousands of reps each day. She performs this explosively.

People generally agree that the majority of females want a great ass. Most woman says that an ass is to a girl is what biceps are to a guy. All girls want a harder, better-rounded behind.

Female physique
If your legs are muscular or big, doing weight-training exercises will make them bigger. Running sprints will develop muscular legs. To reduce the muscular mass in your legs, participate in long-distance running. Arthur Jones proved that long-distance runners have skinny legs. Data proves that long-distance running is the ideal exercise for reducing your lower body mass.

Long distance runners always have skinny, almost shapeless legs that don't even look firm. You do not want that.

262

After you lose some bulk, you can work on bodybuilding or sprint to shape your legs.

If you are attempting to increase your leg size, do high-intensity, short-duration activities. If you are exercising for smaller thigh muscles, the opposite is true. If your objective is to slim your lower body down, make sure to participate in low-intensity, long-duration exercise every day. Those trainees looking to increase their leg size need to predominantly do high-intensity, short-duration activities. I totally believe that long-distance running is the perfect activity for eating away your lower body mass.

When you take a set to the point of brief muscular failure, it forces your body to attempt to find out how to make the task easier the next time. The way your body does this is by building larger muscles. This is not what you want if your lower body is too thick. The key to lower body size reduction is to stay away from the combination of heavy resistance, high volume, and training to failure.

Leg training program:

Exercise	Sets	Reps	Rest
A) Stepmill or Incline Treadmill	1	5 minutes, fast pace	None
B1) Lunge Jumps	3	16 (8 per leg)	None
B2) Squat Jumps	3	8	None
B3) Bodyweight Squats	3	20	60 seconds

Then do long-distance running. This is the perfect activity for eating away your lower body mass. Long distance runners almost always have skinny legs. Now, I'm going to show you the way to a steely, curvaceous ass. Which female athletes have the best ass? That's easy: sprinters!

ASS

Most women want the same thing: a first-class ass.

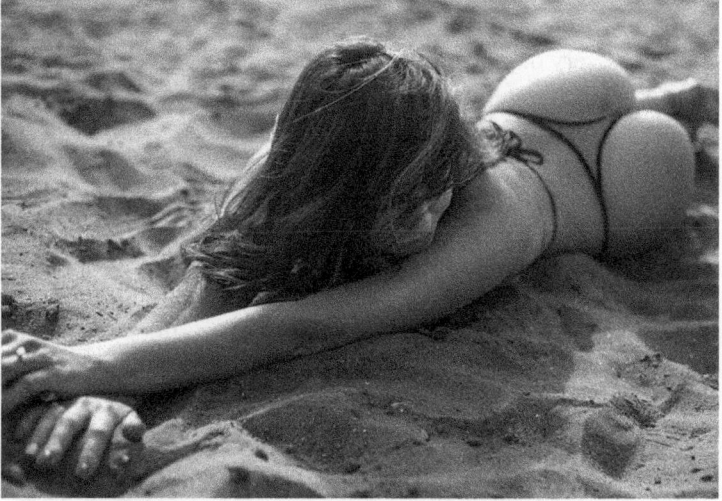

In reality, every girl wants a firmer, shapelier ass. That's no surprise. Everybody knows this. Female young and middle-aged housewives, models, athletes, and movie stars all want the same thing: a great ass.

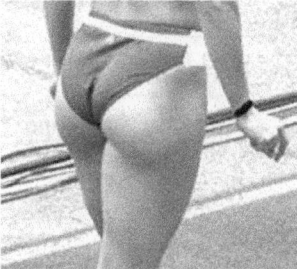

If you ask 20 women which body part they're most interested in developing, chances are at least 19 of them will say, "I want a better butt!"
The truth is, every girl wants a firmer, shapelier ass. Everybody knows this.

The best athletes with top-notch asses are, without a doubt, the sprinters. If you ask, which female athletes have the best ass? That's simple: sprinters!

I believe 100% that training explosively like a sprinter will develop and firm your ass. You know why marathon runners don't develop great ass? because they're not training with enough intensity to work all of the muscle fibers.

Sexy Glutes

What do you think is going to happen to your glutes if you sit all day at a job?

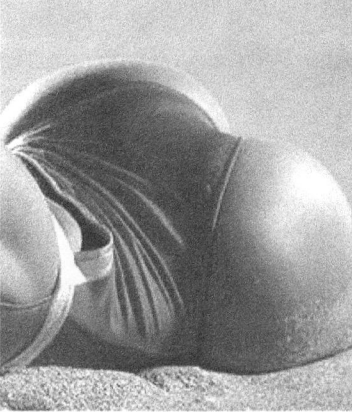

Glutes muscles are a part of your lower body's strength and development. A muscular posterior is also essential for symmetry and, of course, appearance. What comes to mind? Jeans, bikinis, shorts. mini-skirts.
Every woman and man should include exercises for the glutes in every training routine.
You must work your lower body. No way out. The exercises described here will improve your glutes. As you progress, try to do more reps or more sets.

1-Hip Raise

In your back, bend your knees and keep your feet flat on the floor. Lift your hips, hold them for 5 seconds, and then return to their original position. Do 1 set of 12 reps, adding more sets as you progress later on.

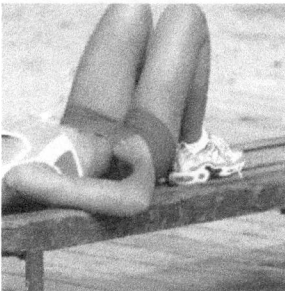

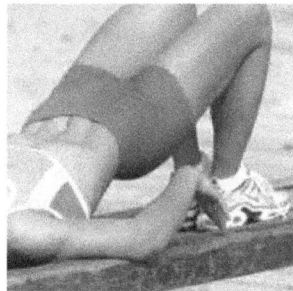

2-Leg back kick

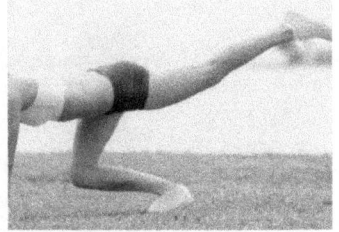

Down in your hands and knees,
maintain a straight back, and extend
one leg behind you. Hold the position
for a few seconds, then return to the
original position. Do one set of 10
reps, change legs and repeat. Add more sets as you progress later on.

3- Lateral Walk

Step to the side, sidestep to the right, keep moving sideways to about
15 feet, then come back sideways to the starting point. Repeat the
process in the opposite direction.

Do 10 reps, adding more sets as you progress later on.

4-Step-up

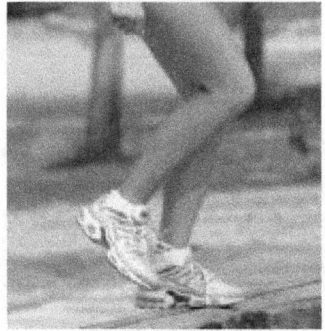

Step up one foot onto a bench or
small table about 4 inches in front
of you.
Return your foot to the floor. Up
and down, alternating between the
right and left foot. Up and down.

5-Medicine ball swing

Grasp a medicine ball
with both hands and
swing it between your
legs, with your knees
bent, down and up, as if
you were chopping wood.

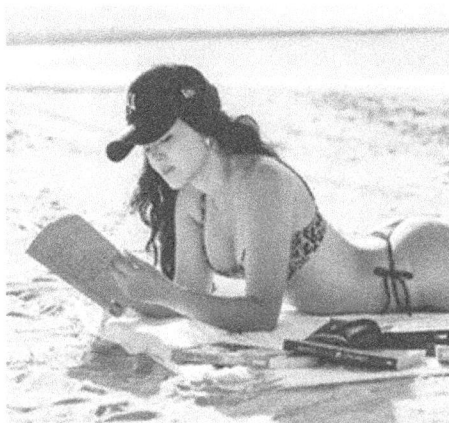
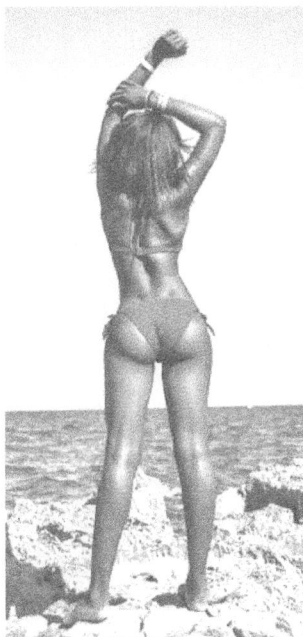
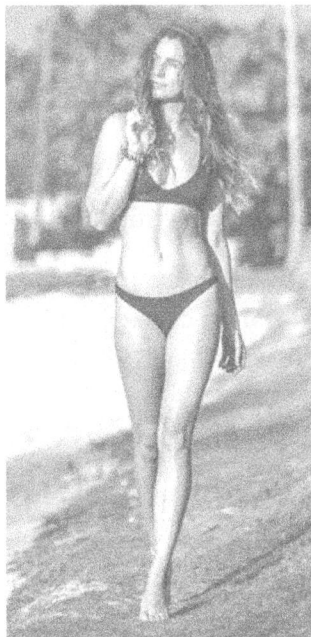

Look great in a bikini

These exercises will make you look sexier and also give you carved-out, powerful glutes. Nice glutes and hamstrings will make you look great in a bikini, and you will be the envious of other girls. Females should avoid exercises that build up the traps, waist, and thighs unless they are very skinny girls with very skinny thighs.

Glutes

Do the next warm-up before the workouts:

Jog in place for 75 strides.

Exercises

Females should avoid exercises for the traps, the waist, and heavy exercises for the thighs. Now the story is different. If you have very skinny thighs, you will want to make them bigger.

Big traps

You should avoid shrugs or any type of upright row with a heavy weight.

Waist

Keep away from Exercises that thicken the waist.

Side bend, particularly with heavier weights, the most damaging things you can do to screw up your middle. Directly abdominal work is unnecessary. Heavy or high volume side bends will make your waist bigger!

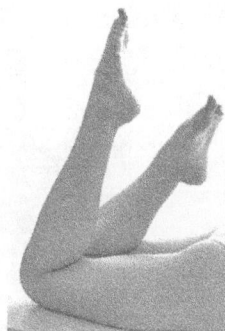

Thighs

Evade: big quads

You should avoid full squat. Full squats will make your thighs and ass bigger.

Skinny girls look good in clothes, but fit chicks look good naked
Ronda Rousey

Waist

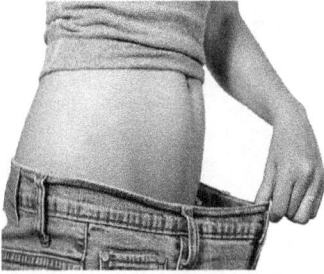

Exercises that thicken the waist ,such as side bends, Doing heavy-weight crunches and side bends will make your waist bigger. Stay away from those.

Thigh Trimming

Losing muscle in just one region of the body, like the thigh, is a hard thing to accomplish, but if you work hard at it, it can be done. The secret to decreasing your body mass is just doing the opposite of what you normally do to build muscles.

Long-distance runners almost always have skinny thighs; you can use this information to reduce your lower body mass a little bit. Stay away from *full* squats and forward lunges. Those exercises can bulk up your thigh muscles.

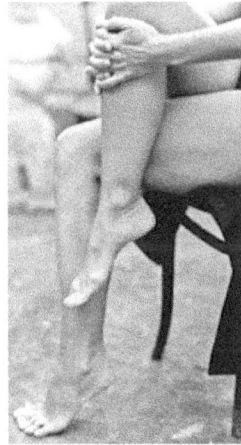

What to Do

Here are two exercises for ass-building workout. You must do them three times per week to get the ass you have always wanted to have. These exercises allow you to contract the gluteus maximus with greatest force.

1. Sprints

How to do it: Run at top speed for 10 seconds.

Exercise Instruction: Perform 6 sprints with one minute of rest between each run.

2. Swings

How to do it: Stand with a wider-than-shoulder-width stance and hold a dumbbell or kettlebell between your legs with both hands.

Squat down until the dumbbell or kettlebell you're holding is below knee level.

Explosively swing the dumbbell, kettlebell, or medicine up to chest height while keeping your arms straight.

Keeps the swinging/squatting action going for 10 seconds. It's essential that you maximally squeeze your glutes (lock out your hips) with each swing. You have here all the tools you need to carve out glutes of granite. You will you look sexier and stronger. Just sprint, swing, and build that ass!

I think that female track and field athletes have some of the sexiest legs and glutes on the planet.

Well-developed glutes and hamstrings are important elements for most women's bodies. No matter if your goal is to win a figure competition or to look great in a bikini, a solid program will get you there faster and more effectively.

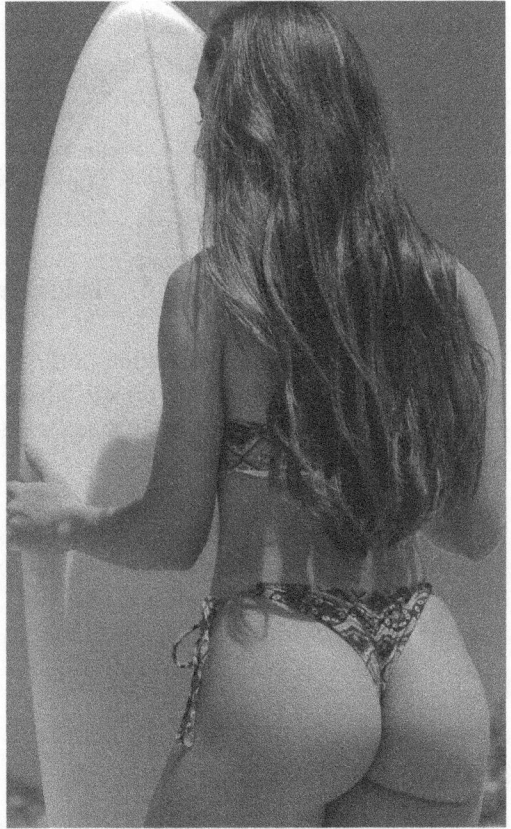

Woman's Core Muscles

Muscle burn more calories than fat.

Strong core muscles perform as your body's main source of power and balance.

The zone between the abdominal and back muscles in the center is the core of the body.

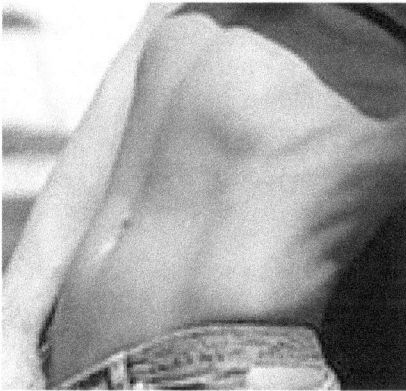

You must develop strength and flexibility in this area so it offers brace and balance, plus it gives you a lean, flat stomach.

The more muscle mass you have, the more calories you'll burn during the day. If you would like to get in shape, strength training is a must.

Strength training works best when it's combined with cardiovascular exercises.
Do cardio exercises to maintain a healthy weight, healthy lungs, and a strong heart.

Do some stretching to keep your muscles long and lean, and to reduce the risk of injury, and help maintain body balance.

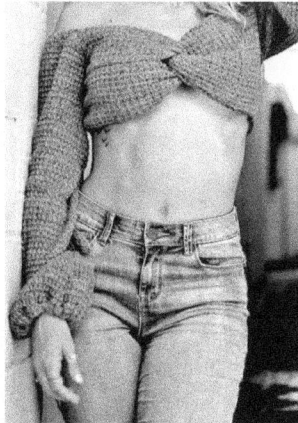

You have to have fear in order to have courage.
Ronda Rousey

Spot Reducing

Don't kill yourself doing 100 sit-ups a day. There is no such thing as spot reducing. You have to lose the fat with aerobics and dieting. Then and only then will your abdominal muscles show.

The object of losing weight is to lose fat without reducing lean tissue. That's hard to do, but harder to maintain. This is increased with training. Forget the scale, look at the mirror.

Scales are useful only to give us a general idea. You don't need a scale to find out you're fat.

The perfect scale is your own image in the mirror. Your waistline will tell you if you are fat. Your weight could be muscle.

You could be 170 pounds with a 34" waist or you could be 170 pounds with a 40" waist.

Many years ago, I learned that when doing exercises, you should focus on the muscle group you are training. You should focus on what you're doing. I have taught people about the mind-body connection and how to concentrate while exercising.

Here is the truth how to lose weight

The word diet originally comes from the Greek word "diaita", which means "manner of living". Here is the truth about how to lose weight. Eat fewer calories by eating less fat and burning more calories by exercising. In the stone age, men killed for their meat, hunting for days and days, many times walking for miles cross-country. They had to work hard just to eat. When was the last time you worked hard for dinner?

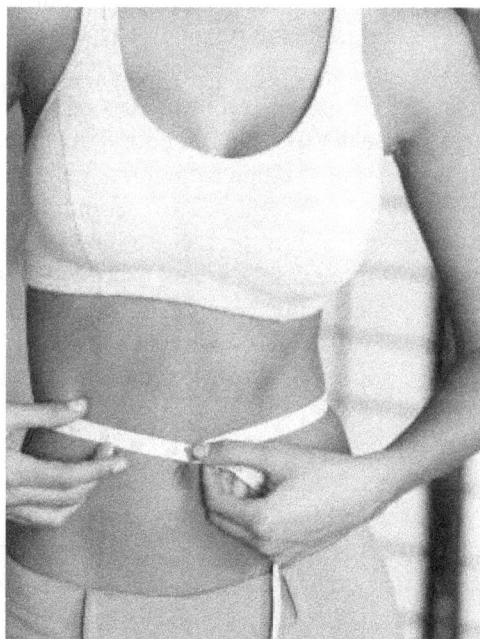

The consumption of meat, poultry, and fish by Americans went up from 165 lbs in the 1920's to 230 lbs. in 2005. Experts say that Americans are eating about 535 more calories per day than they did in 1970.

Every day, 1/3 of children in America eat at a fast food restaurant. 8% of Americans eat at McDonalds every day. They consume 51 pounds of French Fries, and consume about 600 million Big Macs a year and 20 billion hotdogs.

Forty percent of American adolescent girls do not eat any grains at all. 16.9 pounds of potato chips are eaten each year. 35% of Americans are overweight and 26% are obese. Therefore, about two out of three people are overweight. Obesity is defined as being overweight by 20% or more of your desired weight, increasing the risk of many diseases like diabetes, heart disease, and strokes. No wonder there are so many diets and exercise gimmicks today.

The rules for losing weight are simple: eat fewer calories than you burn. Spread calories over several meals throughout the day. When it comes to weight control, exercise can only take you so far.

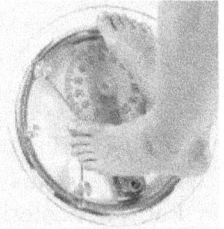

You have to combine both, diet and exercise. The calories you should eat depend on whether you want to lose or gain weight.

According to the American Heart Association, to find out your ideal weight, you should multiply your weight in pounds by (13).

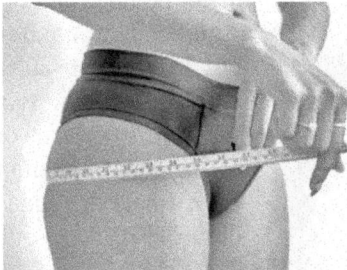

If you want to lose then subtract 250 calories, 55 % of your daily calories should come from complex carbohydrates, 25 % from fat and 15% from protein, sodium intake not more than 3 grams a day. Stick with lean cuts, beans, fish, chicken, vegetables, and plenty of water. Keep track of your calorie intake, and burn off as much as you can by exercising.

Keep in mind that light salad dressing is too heavy on sugar and salt and not too nutritious. Avoid canned food and frozen entrees. Never mix carbohydrates with fats; the key is to eat enough so you don't feel hungry. Don't forget, people that eat 4 or 5 small servings a day lose up to 70% more weight than those that eat 3 big meals a day.

People get confused with the idea of losing fat and losing weight. First you must lose fat, and then you lose weight.

In December 2003, German researchers concluded that water consumption increases the rate at which people burn calories. Doctors from Berlin's Franz-Volhard Clinical Research Center found that men and women burned more calories after drinking about 17 ounces of water. Calorie burn increased by 30% for both men and women.

The researchers also estimate that over a year, a person who increases their water consumption by 1.5 liters a day would burn an extra 17,000 calories, or a weight loss of approximately five pounds. More studies are needed to clearly confirm this weight loss. Remember, never mix carbohydrates with fats and get no sugar from fruits.

Women Training

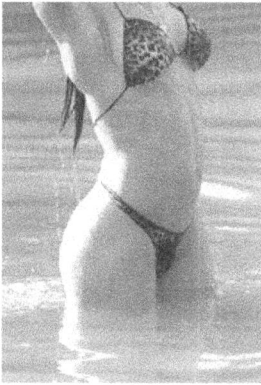

Most women don't like to train hard because they think they will gain men's like muscular bodies. Women have much less testosterone than men do. A woman with normal hormones will always appear feminine, so it's almost impossible to get as much muscle as men do.

Workouts will only help her by improving her complete look. The cosmetic training effects will make her legs firmer, her waist smaller, etc. When exercising and training, I think a woman should concentrate in staying trim, flexible, attractive, sexy and healthy.

Obviously, the method is different, but the basic exercises are the same. You may attain this kind of body by doing cardio exercises like jogging, walking, and stretching to keep yourself flexible, young-looking, and your cardiovascular system in top condition.

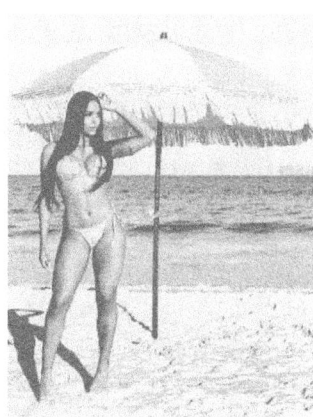

You will certainly lift your bust, get attractive shoulders, gain some lean body weight, or if are overweight, lose it.

Use light or medium weights to obtain toned, strong legs and arms, where women develop problems, particularly under the arms.

After working out and dieting for a couple of months, it's time to recognize your achievements.

Here are ways to treat you.

Go ahead, you deserve it:

Splurge at a spa: Soothe your muscles with 15 relaxing minutes in the steam room; take a long soak in the tub; or go all out and have a long massage.

Go shopping and buy something you've always wanted. Pick out an outfit that shows off your new figure or invest in new workout gear or equipment.

Indulge a little: Have the chocolate cake, or some strawberries and a glass of champagne. Remember, life is not about deprivation.

Information:

Limit your alcohol.

According to the National Cancer Institute, alcohol increases the risk of breast cancer.

Botox is a protein generated by the bacterium Botulinum and is the single most prevalent procedure in the United Estates when injected. Botox works by temporarily reducing wrinkles in the face muscles. So it appears to be smooth. It has both advantages and disadvantages.

Note: being too thin ages your face, according to researchers ta Case Western Reserve University School of Medicine.

Everyone's dream can come true if you just stick to it and work hard.
Serena Williams

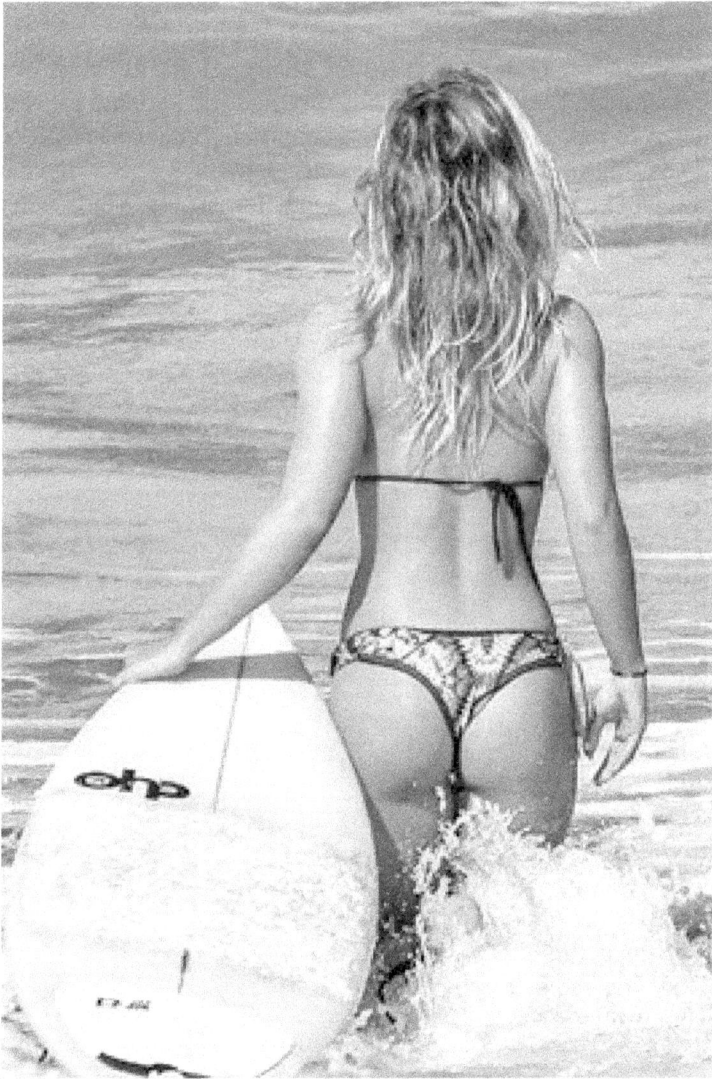

Look great at the beach!

Sprints

Sprints are a long-lost training tool that can develop your conditioning, burn down body fat, and develop a killer set of hamstrings. Walk back the same distance you sprinted for rest between reps. Sprinting places an enormous and unique stress on the hamstrings, glutes, and hips. The acceleration part is where you'll actually be working your glutes and hamstrings as you accelerate to your top speed.

Take a look at the legs of any sprinter, and you will understand what sprinting can do for your legs! The purpose here is hamstring development. If you haven't sprinted in a while, start slow. Intervals are in many ways superior to traditional steady-state training.

Looking hot in a bikini feels incredible, and looking sexy is what being a figure athlete is all about.

If you are female, avoid exercises that build up the traps, waist, and thighs. How you can measure your effort?

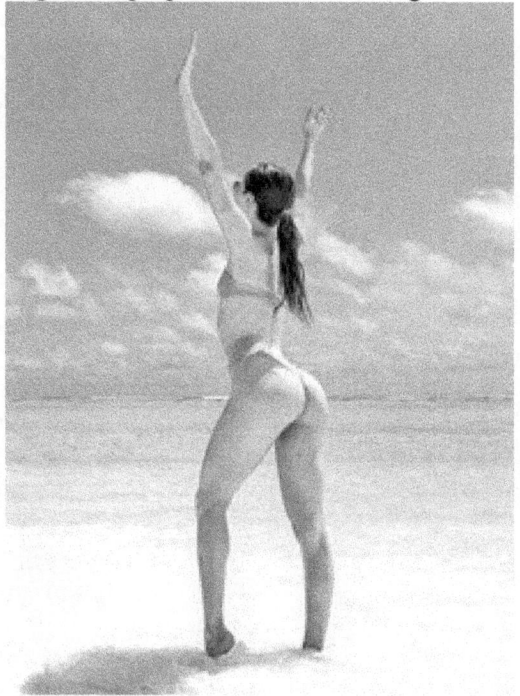

80% of your max speed - fast runs.
90% of your max speed - a very fast run.
95% of your max speed - running very fast.

Traps-Avoid: Big traps. Shrugs and any type of exercise that requires you to upright row a heavy weight.

Exercises that thicken the waist should be avoided.

The exercises you should avoid:
Are there any types of side bends? Doing a bunch of side bends, especially with heavier weights, is one of the worst things you can do to screw up your middle. Most direct abdominal work is unnecessary to develop a bikini body; in fact, it often does more harm than good.

Crunches make me lean.
Not doing endless sets of crunching makes you lean.

Thighs
What we're trying to avoid: big quads, especially the lower, medial portion (the inside of the knee).
These are the exercises you should avoid: full squats and forward lunges. Those exercises can bulk up the muscle that's medial to your knee joint.

Thigh Trimming

Losing fat in one area of the body is difficult. But it can be done. The solution to reducing your lower body is to do the opposite of what develops muscle. It is proven that higher training intensities lead to hypertrophy, if the weight is heavy enough. Ideal for your upper body, but the opposite for your lower body if your intention is to reduce it.

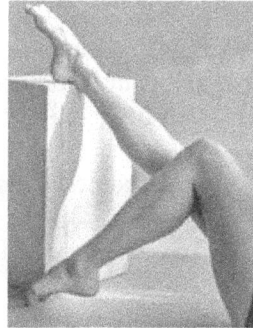

To lower body size, stay away from heavy resistance, high volume, and training to failure. Exercises for reducing legs size:

Incline Treadmill   8 minutes-fast/medium pace
Long distance running   8 to 10 minutes

Fact:
Long distance runners almost always have skinny legs.

Spot reduction is largely a myth.
You probably think these exercises are easy. As you progress and add sets, you will see and feel the difference. By that same time, you will have a very tight and firm buttock.

Skinny calves
Are you worried about wearing shorts because of skinny calves? Try strength training that focuses on the legs. You must work the gastrocnemius (calf) muscles while focusing on the quadriceps (the front of the thighs), hamstrings (back of the thighs), and glutes (buttocks). All are important for strength and leg health.

Your legs include some of the largest muscle groups in your body. Exercising them can help make the most of your ability to burn calories, which means you'll burn more calories all day long, even while resting. In addition, you'll have a leaner, shapelier leg, which will make you look good in shorts.

Calf Raises and Toe-Ups
Focus: calves
Stand with your feet wide apart; keep one hand on a wall or bench for balance. Rise up onto your toes and hold for two to five seconds. Lower yourself to the starting position. Repeat 10 to 20 times. Now flex your feet, raising your toes off the ground so you're standing on your heels; hold for two to five seconds. Repeat 10 to 20 times.

Calisthenics: This is an excellent cardiovascular workout you can do anywhere.
Do each exercise for 25 seconds, then move onto the next one.

Jumping jacks	Push-ups
Jump rope (rope is optional)	Plank reach out
Burpees	

Do this circuit three to five times without any rest. You probably assume it is easy. On the contrary, this circuit will defy many trained folks.

Squats

Start in a standing position. Go down into a squat, come up again, and repeat without pausing.

Jumping Jacks

In a standing position, with feet shoulder-width apart, maintain your arms at your sides. Jump into a wide stance as you bring your arms up overhead. Return to the start in a smooth movement, and repeat without pausing

High Knees

Lift your knees and alternate legs in a running motion, raising the knees high in this fashion each time. in the same way as jogging in place. Sometimes I touch the right elbow with the left knee, alternating right and left.

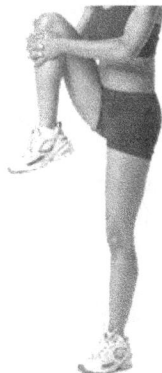

Burpees
Starting in a standing position, squat down; kick your legs back, into a pushup, jump the legs back into a crouch; burst up into a jump, letting the feet leave the ground. When you land, go back into a crouch position and repeat the movement without pausing. This is a killer drill that will get you in shape in no time. Go slowly at the beginning-it is very hard.

Plank reach out
Start with your forearms in a plank position, with elbows under your shoulders, hands facing forward so your forearms are parallel to the floor, and legs extended straight behind you. From this position, reach your right hand and tap the floor in front of you. Return your hand and reach forward with your left hand, tapping the floor in front of you. Continue alternating sides; make sure your back and legs are straight. If it is too hard, place your feet wider apart. The wider the feet, the easier the exercise should be.

What Should You Eat to Lose Belly Fat?

What types of food should you eat to lose weight around your midsection?

Fat that accumulates around the vital organs and around the mid-section is known as visceral fat.

To lose weight in the belly area, you should go on a diet with fruits, vegetables, lean protein, low-fat dairy, whole grains, and reduce portion sizes.

To lose one to two pounds per week, reduce your caloric intake every day. Exercise every day or every two days, aerobically and with weights, for 30 to 60 minutes at a time.

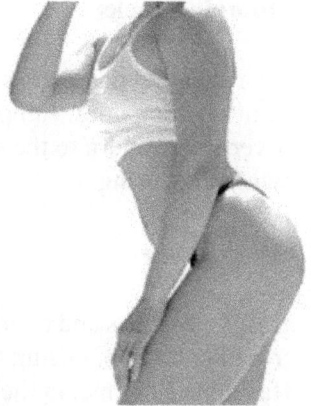

Remember, abdominal exercises won't help you lose fat from the belly area; they'll just tone it. Think about it and do the math. If you eliminate 500 calories a day, you will lose about one pound a week. A reduction of a pound every week will give you 20 pounds lost in about five months.

Some research believes that most people tend to lose fat in the belly area first, then in other areas. I don't believe this theory; I believe that you lose fat from your belly area last.

Here are some tips for you:

Cut out sweet drinks
Drink plain water and low-fat milk.
Physical activity helps you burn calories while improving your health.
Eat small portions; replace high-calorie foods with low-calorie foods.
Too much time in between meals makes your body go into panic survival mode and start storing fat.
Eat meals every 2.5 to 3 hours.

Eat fiber!

Eating foods with fiber helps maintain your blood sugar at a consistent level.

Consume healthy fats.

Healthy fats help us with fat loss, protecting our muscle mass, supporting energy, and also helping with mental clarity, focus, vitality, and longevity.

Eat an adequate amount of calories.

If you don't plan correctly, you are going fast to find yourself tired, grumpy, and irritable.

Don't eat too many calories.

People do hours of cardio when they don't see the results. They are surprised to find out that the cardio is not working.

Don't deprive yourself!
It's okay to eat a favorite cheat food a couple of times a week. Use good judgment and moderation. Enjoy the process without depriving yourself!

Fat loss techniques
The word diet originally comes from the Greek word "diaita", which means manager of living.

Proper nutrition
Activities that burn calories and elevate metabolism keep burning more calories after the exercise session. According to one study of dieting overweight patients, 83 percent of dieters regained all of the weight they lost.

Another study discovered that 50 percent of dieters gained 11 pounds over their starting weight just five years after starting the diet!

Crash Diets

Crash diets don't work in the long run. You know why? When you restrict your calorie intake, it causes a lot of muscle loss. This puts a stop to your fat-burning metabolism, triggering you to gain all the weight back within months of normal eating.

Dieting Out

1- Do not stuff your face

2 - Order a Salad- No dressing is best, with the exception of an oil and vinegar mix.

3-Order Clean-grill chicken breasts, fish, or a lean cut of beef.

4-Portion control: A restaurant gives you more than you should have.

5- Have a Cheat Meal -An occasional meal at your favorite restaurant

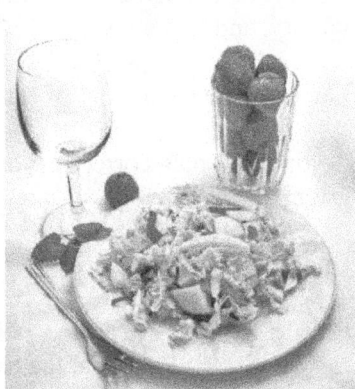

The truth about losing weight

The rules for losing weight are simple: eat fewer calories and burn more by exercising. In the stone age, men killed for their meat, hunting for days and days, many times walking for miles cross-country. They had to work hard just to eat. When was the last time you worked hard to eat?

Experts declare that Americans eat 535 more calories per day than they did in 1970. Forty percent of American teenagers do not eat any grains at all.35% of Americans are overweight and 26% are obese. Obesity is described as being overweight by 20% more of your appropriate weight, raising the risk of many complaints like diabetes, heart disease, and strokes.

Consume lean cuts, beans, fish, chicken, vegetables, and plenty of water. Watch your calorie intake and burn off calories by exercising.

Evade canned food and frozen entrees. Never mix carbohydrates with fats; the key is to eat a sufficient amount so you don't feel hungry.

People get confused with the thought of losing fat and losing weight. Initially, you must lose fat, and then you lose weight.

In December of 2003, German researchers determined that drinking water increases the rate at which individuals burn calories. Doctors from Berlin's Franz-Volhard Clinical Research Center discovered that men and women burned more calories after drinking about 17 ounces of water. Calorie burn was boosted by 30% for both men and women.

The researchers also calculated that over a year, a person who increases his water consumption by 1.5 liters a day would burn an extra 17,000 calories, or an estimated five pounds. More investigations are needed to clearly authenticate this weight loss.

Dining out

Cut your meal in half.

Dining out is a big problem for overeating because of the large portion sizes many restaurants serve. When you go out, eat only half of your meal.

Splitting a dish with a friend is another easy and cost-effective way to eat less. Sometimes I do that with my wife.

Slow Down/Enjoy

Most people are used to rushing, so we rush even when eating. When you eat fast, you normally eat too much. Another mistake is eating while watching TV or surfing the Internet. It's more likely you'll overeat. I never eat while washing the TV. This is a no-no in my home.

<u>Consume Water</u>

You have to drink fewer high-calorie beverages or stop drinking them.

Social Networking: If you can't recruit a buddy in the flesh, try connecting with a cyber friend. The Internet provides more opportunities to meet a buddy with similar fitness goals, and online diet groups are an ideal way to share your experiences with other dieters, get support, and celebrate your successes without a major time commitment.

Here are four ways to break free from your weight-loss routine:

Try a new food or cuisine every week. Japanese, Chinese, Indian, and Greek cuisine all have healthy options. Add walnuts and yogurt to cereal and salads, and use high-quality olive oil instead of canola or peanut oil to fry food.

Don't constantly eat turkey on whole wheat; try a soup and a salad. Make sure to eat a good portion of veggies like carrot sticks, lettuce, and tomatoes.

Eat with friends; it helps you eat less by chairing a portion or even conversing. Keep yourself motivated.

Cut or Eliminate
Avoid:
Sugars and Flours, Refined Sugar substitutes, saccharin, and cyanide should all be avoided. Such as cookies, pies, cakes, fat

Those found in red meat and unpreserved vegetable oils are the worst.
Frozen Dinners
Processed desserts
Canned Vegetables
Processed Meats -preserved with preservative

Nutrition rules

A) Eat every few hours-Too long in between "meals" is one damaging mistakes many people make.

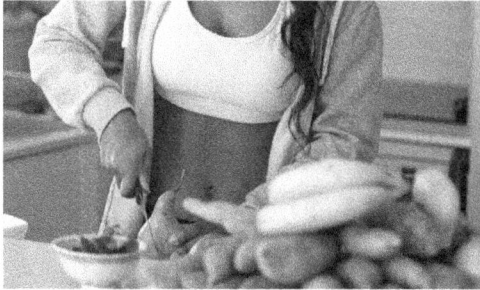

Eating long time between meals makes your body kick into panic-survival mode instead. Instead, eat smaller meals every 2.5 to 3 hours.

B) Consume protein at every meal: This is critical when dieting because calories are limited and muscle can be sacrificed to use energy for recovery.

C) Eat calorie-Be smart when you eat and count calorie intake. If the deprivation is substantial, your body will go into a panic-survival mode. This is prejudicial for dieters because your body gives the order to keep all the calories you take as fat.

D) Not too many calories-Eat the sufficient calories you need.

E) Consume fiber: Consuming fiber foods helps to keep blood sugar levels stable. Go slowly. Your digestive system will need time to get used to the added fiber. Too much gas is often the result of increasing fiber too fast.

F) Consume healthy fats-Consuming healthy fats provides numerous benefits, including increased energy, mental clarity, focus, health, vitality, and longevity! Example: salmon, avocados, olive oil, flaxseeds, and omega oils.

Don't totally deprive yourself!-Have a favorite "cheat" food once or twice a week. Use common sense and moderation.

Easy Foods

There's no need to count calories; just select "clean" foods.
Protein: lean steak, grilled chicken breasts, turkey breast, baked or grilled fish,
Veggies: green veggies, broccoli,
Starch: sweet potato, whole-wheat pasta, etc.

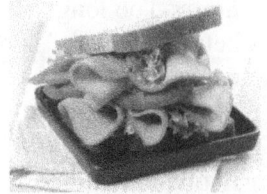

That's it-portion size control and quality food. This is the key to an athletic, sexy, and strong body. Individuals that diet lose weight and also lose muscle along with fat.

Many people do yo-yo dieting, a cycle of weight loss followed by fat gain, followed by more weight loss and then more fat gain. Doctors claim that it takes about 20 minutes for your stomach to "know" it's full. This is why you eat until you're full, and then 20 minutes later you feel completed stuffed.

Dessert: fruit

KIWI- Provide potassium, magnesium, vitamin C, vitamin E, and fiber.

An apple a day keeps the doctor away? Full of antioxidants and flavonoids, they reduce the risks of colon cancer, heart attack, and stroke.

Strawberries are full of antioxidants.

Eating 2-4 oranges a day helps keep colds out, decreases cholesterol.

Guava and papaya are rich in fiber and help prevent constipation.

"Learning never exhausts the mind."
Leonardo da Vinci

Cellulite

"Cellulite! This word makes women shiver. Cellulite is only fat, which appears usually on the thighs and buttocks and creates the appearance of cottage cheese. All women hate it. Cellulite builds up mostly in women. If you are fat, it increases your chances of getting cellulite, but numerous women who are slim get it too.

Strategies and Suggestions

Size-Lose weight and keep an eye on the calories you take every day.

Exercise: Exercise will help you reduce body fat, including cellulite.

Surgery: Some people have had liposuction procedure, but this will not work all the time.

So what causes this gruesome condition? Cellulite is simply bumps of fat leaked through weakened tissue that has split up from the skin, generating bulges that have a denser, harder feel to them. Generally, people believe that cellulite is the result of fatness. This is not true; this condition affects everyone, from fashion models to the average working class female, to mothers, and even athletes.

Cellulite is not a disease, but it is very disturbing to those who are touched by it. Cellulite has prevented millions of females from participating in many activities, like going to the beach.

Most women get cellulite, as well as thin women. Specialists affirm that about 80 percent of women over age 18 have cellulite. There are numerous creams advertised for this problem, but there is currently no cure. 95% of women have some cellulite on their bodies. Very rarely does it appear in men. It is extremely difficult for a woman to attain and keep a lean, trim body. Remember to eat balanced meals, four or five small portions, and eat early in the evening. Also, a good idea is to stay away from the sun or use sun protection.

Cellulite loves:

Setting around
Processed & refined foods
Caffeine
Alcohol

Cellulite hates:

Exercise
Low fat diet
Lots of water

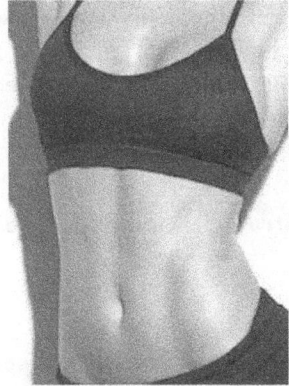

Sexy trim, lean waist

There are some foods with natural diuretic properties that will help you decrease fluid buildup. Some of these are asparagus, parsley, cranberries, apple cider vinegar, and caffeine.

Also, a good source of nutrients comes from fatty fish, in the form of omega-3 fatty acids. Omega-3 fatty acids increase your circulation and lower your blood pressure.

Also helps the anti-cellulite fight inflammation. Omega-3 fats, together with the alpha linolenic acid found in flaxseed, are the most powerful anti-inflammatory fats available to us.

One fruit you should add to your fight in the anti-cellulite battle is pineapple. It possesses an enzyme called bromelain.

It has been confirmed that this substance helps in reducing water retention and, at the same time, is a natural anti-inflammatory agent.

You can find many anti-cellulite creams on the market, but there is no scientifically proven way to reduce cellulite at all.
Some experts believe cellulite is inefficient circulation in the area and, lastly, inflammation.

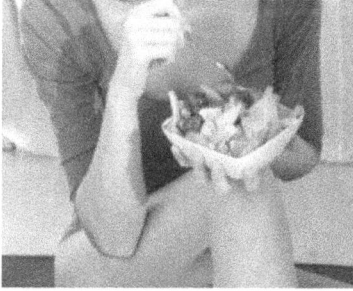

Diuretic properties Natural foods will decrease fluid buildup, which will help you keep the skin smooth.

These are celery, cranberries, parsley, asparagus, apple cider vinegar, and caffeine. Include several of these into your meal strategy to get extra help.

Onions and garlic have been revealed to improve circulation and help lower blood pressure. Studies show that if taken regularly, these nutrients will also lead to a strong heart and a longer, healthier life.

Another source of help you can get is from the fruit pineapple. It has an enzyme called bromelain. This substance is helpful in lowering water retention, edema, and bruising, and at the same time promotes healing and is a natural anti-inflammatory agent.

This is the plan of attack in your war against cellulite. Keep it up; exercise, watch what you eat, and you will get a bikini body.

Rules for Nutrition

1) Eat every few hours; skipping meals is the worst thing a person can do to lose weight. It makes your body kick into panic survival mode and store fat in case it is needed later on. Instead, eat smaller meals every 2.5 to 3 hours.

2) Consume protein

It is important when dieting, because calories are being restricted and you will lose muscle.

3) Consume fiber

Foods high in fiber will help keep your blood sugar at a consistent level, which means you're less likely to crave junk food.

4) Healthy fats

Foods like salmon, walnuts, avocados, olive oil, flaxseeds, and omega oils will help you with fat loss, protecting your muscle mass, energy production, mental clarity and focus, vitality, and longevity!

5) Consume calories

Under-eating too much, or waiting too long to eat, will hinder your results. Your body will go into panic-survival mode. Everything you eat, your body will store as fat. You will be unmotivated to work out, tired, grumpy, irritable, and fail to see the results you are after.

6) Excessive calorie consumption

Keep an eye on your calorie intake.

7) Reward day

One day a week, eat anything you want, go out with a friend or a date, and order a pizza or a drink. Just don't overdo it, use common sense and moderation. It's easier to keep a healthy diet this way.

Yogurt: it's alive!

Yogurt with active cultures. These cultures, or active bacteria, support digestion, keeping your belly happy. Yogurt is one of the dairy products that can assist you in fighting lactose intolerance because of the natural presence of lactase, an enzyme that helps digest lactose.

Spinach: The Green Giant

Spinach has many benefits for both men and women. In women, benefits range from bone health to fighting ovarian cancer. This is a green that's filled with all you need to help build your muscles in a balanced diet. Spinach has the ability to help transport oxygen from the lungs to the muscles, where it can be stored.

Bananas:

This fruit can replenish your potassium, stores, which is essential for electrolytes, balance.

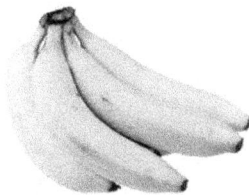

A banana is loaded with potassium. If you eat one pre-workout, it will help you with muscle contractions during exercise. The sugar helps with protein delivery and glycogen into your muscles.

Findings have indicated that fish oil helps fight joint stiffness and muscle fatigue.

Turkey: Turkey protein boosts natural metabolic, selenium, and vitamin B6 levels.

Broccoli: delivers a good supply of vitamin C.

Water: Drink lots of water! It keeps you hydrated and keeps yours system flushed.

Pregnant

When my mother was pregnant, the doctor advised her not to do anything. She had to stay in bed most of the time. Things are different now, and doctors recommend some kind of exercise.

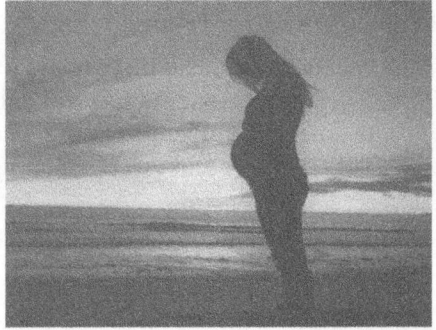

You should always check first with your doctor. Everybody is different. Your training should be low-impact, like walking, swimming, and only with your doctor's approval. Don't push yourself, follow your doctor's recommendation, and remember that this is a beautiful time and you will always have time later on. Learn how to eat, exercise, and care for yourself.

You gave birth: You gave birth to a perfect boy or girl after much anticipation, and your big task now is to find out if you can get your body back. Of course you can. Start working out a little by little in the short training section. Keep adding exercises and time working out, and in a couple of months, you will look amazing!

Exercising while Dieting

1 – Don't eat too much like there's no tomorrow.
2 – Request a salad with only the oil and vinegar mixture as dressing.
3 – Select from grilled chicken breasts, fish, or a lean cut of beef.
4 – Portion control: always leave some food on the plate.
5): Once in a while, treat yourself to a cheat meal with some friends.

If you want to have a kid in the future, you'll need to know how to diet and exercise so that you have the best chance of having a healthy pregnancy and losing weight afterward. Ask your waiter if you don't see some kind of food on the menu; ask if they can accommodate you

Muscle burns more calories than fat

An active person with muscle mass burns more calories sitting than a sedentary person with fewer muscles.

Ways to Burn Fat at Home

Chopping Wood	Gardening
Mowing the Lawn	Laying Carpet or Tile
Shoveling Snow	Walking the dog
Moving Furniture	Cleaning the family car
Painting the House	Unloading Groceries
Light House Cleaning	

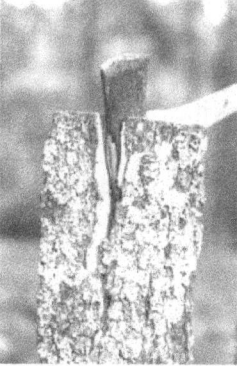

Chopping wood

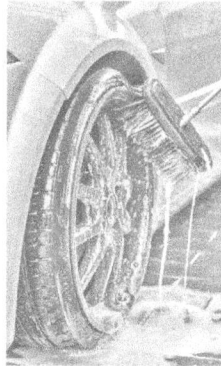

cleaning car

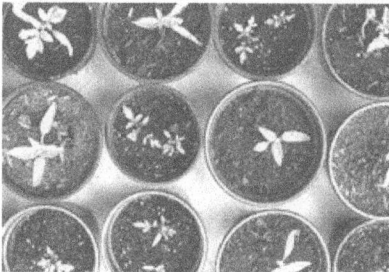

Gardening

Calorie-Expenditure Chart

Calories per minute

Calories burned per minute of activity

Running quickly	8.90
Swimming fast	8.00
Weight training	8.00
Cycling	7.60
Walking fast	3.20
Walking easily	.85

This list is only an approximation. I'm including it as a guide to your physical activity.

CALORIE COUNT

Calorie use in 30 min. activities

Activity	Calories use
Aerobics	210
Cycling	120
Slowly Jogging	270
Swimming	283
Rowing Machine	210

These activities were calculated for a person weighing 160 lbs. So it will vary up or down from person to person. Use only as a guide to figure out how many calories you'll burn doing any of them.

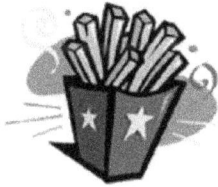

Fast Foods

Subway

Veggie delight 1

Turkey breast 1

Turkey breast & ham 1

Subway club 1

Roasted chicken breast 1

Water 8 oz

Burger King

Chicken sandwich 1

Chicken whopper 1

Whopper Jr. 1

Whopper- (take out the bread) 1

Chicken nuggets 8

Diet soda (small glass)

Water 8 oz

McDonald's

Chicken sandwich grilled 1

Chicken sandwich 1

Salad 1

Big Mac (take the bread out) 1

Chicken nuggets

Orange juice 8 oz

Diet soda (small glass)

Water 8 oz

Wendy's

Chicken sandwich 1

Chicken salad 1

Green salad 1

Diet soda (small glass)

Water 8 oz

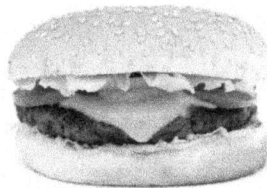

Diet-Sample

A Sample of Muscle weight gain

Breakfast

- 2-Eggs
- Boiled
- Poached
- Orange juice
- Coffee
- Cereal
- Milk
- Bread
  Turkey
- Protein drink
- Light meat
- Fruit
- Cottage cheese
- water

Mid-Morning
- Milk
- Shake

Lunch
- Light Meat
- Turkey
- Cottage Cheese
- Tuna
- Chicken
- Sandwich of the above

Dinner
- Grilled Meat
- Salad
- Grilled Veal
- Soup
- Bread

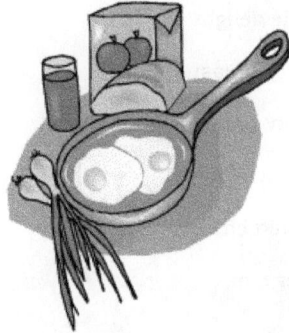

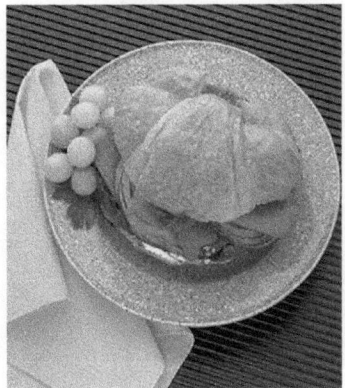

Sample Lose Weight

Breakfast
2-Eggs: Boiled
Poached
Bread no Butter
Coffee no Milk

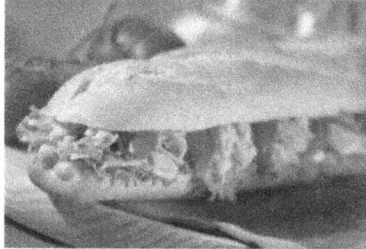

Lunch
Turkey
Chicken Skinless
Canned Tuna Water

Tuna sandwich

Grapefruit
Water
Orange Juice

Dinner
Green Salad
Tomato
Turkey   > Grilled or Broiled
Chicken   > Grilled or Broiled
Veal   >Grilled or Broiled
Water
Skip Salt

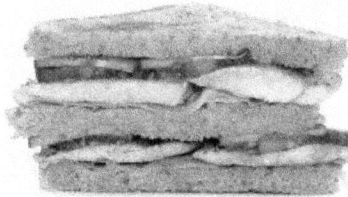

Chicken sandwich

Skip Sodas
Skip frozen foods and fast food restaurants

Lose fat

Here you are aiming to lose flab. Don't go by the scale. Consider how you look in the mirror or how your clothes fit you, rather than how many pounds you've lost. Don't hurry either. Reduce your calorie intake by 500 milligrams per day, spread your calorie intake over several meals, and include cardiovascular exercise two or three times per week. Don't overeat, leave food on your plate, don't have seconds, eat early.

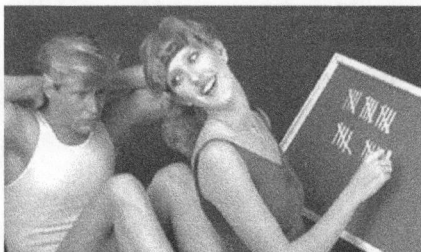

Losing weight is hard, but keeping it off is even harder. Only about 5% of the people who try to lose weight keep it off. I believe heredity plays a very important role in obesity. This does not mean you can't lose weight if you exercise and eat well.

Today, it's a fact that the American population is eating more fat than ever before. Most of us watch TV after dinner, right? So we sit for hours when, in reality, we should be taking a walk around the block for 15 or 20 minutes.

This is a great idea for digestion and for keeping us trimmed. Walk fast, then slowly, listening to your body. Go slow, but get out and <u>do it.</u>

Dancing:

I knew a professional bodybuilder, Sergio Oliva, who was Mr. Universe, Mr. America, and Mr. Olympia. He used to dance a lot and, at the same time, got into incredible shape. Dancing is an amazing workout.

You'll increase stamina and balance –it will help your heart, lungs and your overall stress levels.

Salsa, disco, and rock are all fun and an excellent cardio activity.

Chicken or Turkey Chicken and turkey contain great amount of protein and very low fat. You can eat them grilled, roasted, or broiled. It is much better if you remove the skin; this is where most of the fat is found. White meat turkey has less fat than chicken breast. Try to buy free-range chickens or organic chickens. It is a much better choice because they are free of antibiotics and chemicals.

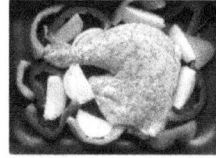

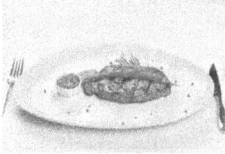

Lean meat is high in protein, B vitamins, B-12 vitamins, iron, zinc, and a variety of other nutrients. Try it. Meats like buffalo and antelope are high in protein and very low in fat, but they are very expensive, try it .Grass-fed beef has less fat, fewer calories and is a much healthier choice. Grass fed cattle has no antibiotics or hormones. I warn you, it is very expensive.

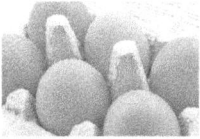

Eggs are inexpensive and provide a high protein source. The Yolk contains a lot of choline. A few years back, doctors recommended people be careful about eating them eggs because they thought they could raise cholesterol. This is not the case anymore. Testosterone is derived from cholesterol. Think about this! You can buy eggs with improved Omega-3's. Also, you can buy organic eggs from chickens that are free from antibiotics and chemicals. It is better if you buy them cage free.

Milk- mature animals don't drink milk. Is this something that we all should know? A glass of milk is full of calcium and is excellent for strong bones and teeth. Dairy products are high in calcium and vitamin D.A better choice is low-fat milk or low fat dairy products. Yogurt is a great choice, but you must be careful with the ones packed with fruit. These are packed with sugar and thickeners. Greek yogurt is an excellent choice.

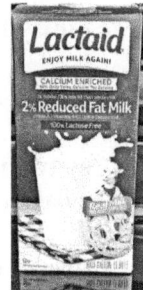

Chew your milk instead of drinking it.

301

Top Sirloin: top of the list for muscle building mass, strength-high in testosterone levels, creatine, and glutamine. Not restricted

Bison meat is loaded with protein to increase muscle mass and strength. It is pricey. Not restricted

Whole eggs: Each has about 8 grams of protein per serving, 3 a day for larger gains in size and strength. It is **proven** that eggs do not **raise cholesterol** in young, active athletes. Not restricted

Chickens-Chicken breast-is a fat free-protein dream. Not restricted

Fish- Lean and high in protein, for maximum mass and strength. Tilapia (Tilapia)-The Red Snapper-Trout Trout

Black beans (not canned) are rich in protein, fiber, and slow digestion. Carbs enhance muscle mass. Not restricted

Whole grain rice: One cup of rice with one cup of black beans contains about the same protein as a 2.5-ounce steak. One cup.

Backed sweet potatoes-Fast digesting carbs it keeps insulin stable and provides energy. One or two per day, early in the day

Day snacks; beef sticks, buffalo stick, chicken sticks. Not limited.

Greek yogurt has no flavor, but contains -18 grams of protein, three times the amount in regular yogurt, one or two a day.

2 pints of ice cream per day, any flavor

8 glasses of water or more per day or no limit

Any two fruits per day, never with dinner or in the evening, early in the day (1 hour or 12 hours before workout).

Bananas are **better**	Apples
Blueberries	Strawberries

We all think eating fruits means just buying fruits. It's important to know how and when to eat. What is the correct way of eating fruits? Some nutritionist recommends not eating fruits after your meals! And that fruits should be eaten on an empty stomach. Not sure? Try it yourself.

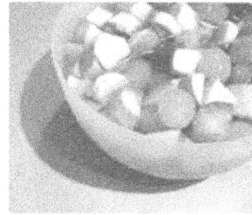

Juices-Orange juice-early in the day-**one cup**

Cranberry (low sugar): to keep the kidneys and the urinary track system clean (early in the day), one glass a day, when you need to drink fruit juice, drink only fresh fruit juice, not juice from cans.

Eating a whole fruit is better than drinking the juice.
If you must drink juice, drink it mouthful by mouthful slowly, for the reason you must let it mix with your saliva before swallowing it.

According to experts, you can go on a 3-day fruit fast to cleanse your body. Just eat fruits and drink fruit juice throughout the 3 days and you will be schoked when your friends tell you how radiant you look!

Supplements

B12 -One dropper a day or one injection shot a week to protect against stress and aid metabolism.

Argentina's Desiccated Liver, vacuum-dried, is an excellent protein supplement for size and mass. A favorite of the Golden Bodybuilding Era champions, one or two a day.

Complete Amino Acids-one or twice a day between meals-(any)

Supplements The 3 day on/2 day off schedule cleans any toxics from the liver, kidneys, and stomach and helps the body use the supplements without getting used to them.

Always eat slowly.

Beer

Beer Boosts Vitamin Levels

Beer contains vitamin B6, B12, and folic acid, and one study discovered that beer drinkers had 30% higher vitamin B6 levels in their blood than non-beer drinkers.

Beer builds stronger bones

They are rich in silicon, a compound that is associated with better bone health.

Heart disease is reduced.

Drinking a pint of beer a day reduces your risk of heart disease, according to an investigation of 16 studies involving more than 200,000 people. However, those who drank more than a pint were at a higher risk for heart disease.

Diabetes is reduced.

According to studies, drinking two beers per day can reduce your risk of type 2 diabetes by 25%.According to various studies, beer increases insulin sensitivity, which helps protect against diabetes.

Lowering blood pressure

Most people by now know that wine is good for your heart, but beer is much better. A study of more than 70,000 women aged 25 to 40 found that those who drank moderate beer daily were less likely to experience high blood pressure than women who drank wine and spirits.

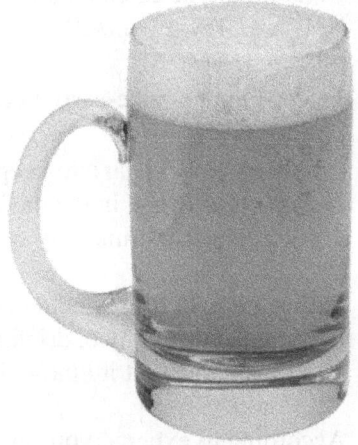

It prevents blood clots.

Again, reports conclude that drinking moderate beer prevents blood clots from forming and obstructing blood flow to the heart, neck, and brain, which can cause a stroke.

It improves brain health.

Drinking one beer per day can reduce the risk of mental decline in older men and women by up to 20%.

It reduces the likelihood of kidney stones

Reports conclude again that men's drinking a bottle of beer daily can lower their risk of getting kidney stones by 40 percent, probably due to beer's high water content of 93 percent.

Life Lengthens

USDA Several studies conclude that beer drinkers tend to live longer. The USDA estimates that moderate drinking prevents about 26,000 deaths a year. The study reports that if European beer drinkers discontinued drinking, there would be a two-year reduction in life expectancy.

Limit alcohol if you are a woman

According to the National Cancer institute, alcohol increases the risk of breast cancer.

Normal aging

When men age, there is a slow decrease in testosterone production. Mature men normally have lower testosterone than younger men do. Keep in mind that the classification of low testosterone levels differs from laboratory to laboratory. Over-all, less than 200 or 250 ng/dL is considered low. Testosterone readings can vary over several days.

Evaluation has to be based on additional measurement. Current findings have established vitamin D3's ability to increase testosterone levels. They also say that vitamin D3 can help fighting fatigue, depression, muscle loss, and pain associated with aging.
To learn more about Vitamin D3, speak with your doctor.

Omega-3s (EPA and DHA)

Omega-3 fat EPA and DHA (found in fish oil) are vital for hormone production together with testosterone. In a diet without fat, the body will not be able to produce testosterone and other hormones. Omega-3s are also anti- inflammatory.

Zinc If you decide to use a zinc supplement, stick to a dosage of less than 40 mg a day.

Impotence -Erectile Dysfunction

Two double-blind, placebo- controlled trials, including a total of about 135 individuals, verify that Korean red ginseng may improve erectile function. In one of the trials, 45 participants took one or the other, placebo or Korean red ginseng at, a dose of 900 mg 3 times daily for 8 weeks.

The conclusions show that while using Korean red ginseng, men experienced much better sexual function than while taking placebos. If you are single and sexually active, you need to use condoms to prevent STIs and unwanted pregnancies. Abstinence is the only way to decrease the risk of STIs.

Nutritional Value

If you eat a three-ounce serving of red meat (beef), it will give you half (about 25g) of your suggested daily protein intake. It is also a great source of vitamins B6 and B12, zinc, and a good source of iron.

Heart Health

Most people believe that red meat increases the risk of coronary disease. An up-to-date report indicates that eating three ounces a day of lean red meat was not related to a higher risk of heart disease or diabetes.

The healthiest cuts of red meat

If you want to eat one of the healthiest cuts of red meat, choose pork tenderloin. It only has approximately 122 calories per serving and is rich in protein and B vitamins.

Staying Younger

According to science, there is a difference between chronological and biological age, which means you might be 46 years old and have the body of a 36-year-old.

Genetics? This is most likely the correct response. Nonetheless, staying and looking young requires a combination of exercise, good sleep, a nutritious diet, and reduced stress.

Booster

Vitamin D2 (Vitamin D2)
Experts claim that Vitamin D2 is cheaply made, and they also claim that the D3 form is much better quality.

Testosterone

According to studies, 60 percent of men over 65 have free testosterone levels that are lower than those of men in their 30s and 35s.

This is what occurs as you get older:

1. Your metabolism decreases, making losing weight very difficult to do.

2. Your hormones, in charge of skin, muscle, and sex drive, start dropping each year.

3. Your memory starts to decline.

4. Bones get weaker.

Evidence: When you exercise, you'll be activating your hormones. So, exercise to stay young!

Sharpen your mind

Stay current on current events.

Sharpen your mind with problem solving situations.

Keep your brain busy.

Maintaining an active mind is as important as staying physically fit.

Keep up with the new modern gadgets

Early to bed and early to rise makes a man healthy, wealthy, and wise.
Benjamin Franklin

Mature
Bodybuilding

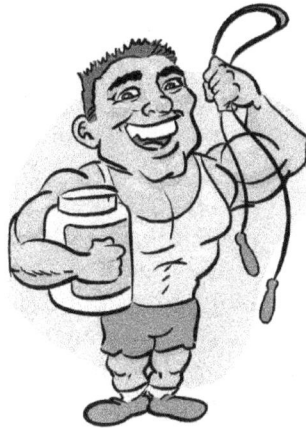

A mature bodybuilder should concentrate on lean body weight. He should make sure he does aerobic exercises two or three times a week to help lower his heart rate, and improves his circulation, and keep his weight down. These must also include stretching exercises. It is important as you age to stay flexible. According to the census bureau, 25 million people are over the age of 65, and by 2030, more than 64 million will be 65 or older.

Your training workouts should be intense and short, and should concentrate on the big muscles like the chest, back, legs, etc. Most people accept age as an excuse for inactivity. Most think they are too old to exercise. Not the baby boomers. They want to keep active and young. This generation does not want to get old. Why would they want to? A young male will rebound much more easily from an injury than an older male, who is going to take much longer to heal.

Fitness is health; health is freedom from disease. Everybody by now knows that exercise is good for your heart. With exercise, the heart becomes stronger and richer in oxygen, and the heart beats slowly at rest and at work. The best exercise is a continuous, rhythmic one, which makes the muscles pump blood repetitively.

Another reason for exercising is longevity. It is proven that people who exercise live longer and healthier, get fewer heart attacks, and if they do get one, it is most likely they will survive it. Mature bodybuilders should choose a body weight for the rest of their lives. If you are under severe emotional stress, take a few days off, don't push so hard, and come back after a few days.

Always warm up and cool down. If you have back problems, swimming is a marvelous activity. Also, pull down on a lat machine, and avoid exercises that compress the spine, such as lifts and presses.

Don't make your program so rigorous that you may get injured. The goal here is to get stronger, lose fat, stay flexible, and be toned. Train, don't strain, and don't bounce the weights. You must stop or reduce smoking and control your alcohol intake; you may choose to bend the rules for an occasional or special event or celebration. Keep an eye on caffeine and salt if you have high blood pressure. Make sure to stand tall, chin in. The price of a faulty posture is loss of height, strain on the spine, a sagging chest and more.

Standing tall can make you look years younger and restore mobility to your body. Two of the major problems of aging are posture and flexibility. When exercising, the moment you feel discomfort, which is the beginning of pain, stop. Another factor in staying young is relaxation. Playing and laughing helps the gastrointestinal system and lowers blood pressure, among other things.

A well-balanced diet is also key. It should include protein, vitamins, minerals, fiber, and lots of water. Minimize sugar and sodium. Try to eat when you are hungry, don't skip meals, exercise every day, and sleep the necessary hours your body needs. As you get older, you need fewer calories to keep going. Exercise increases the filtration of blood through the kidneys and drains fluid in the process. It must be replaced with drinking water, at least ten glasses a day to wash the irritants out.

When I'm talking to people, the age factor always comes up. Again, I'll be honest with you. I never think of aging. When I was in my 40's, I was in much better shape than guys 20 years younger. I've used these concepts throughout my bodybuilding and training years and have remained injury free. I still love to exercise. The thought of exercising still excites me. Of course, I don't work-out as hard as I used to during my younger years and I don't go to my maximum every day.

"A smile will gain you ten more years of life".
Chinese Proverb

MY ARTICLE

Are you too old? Straight-up Talk- the Fountain of Youth

Every time I watch a championship fight and the champion loses or does very poorly, I hear the same old story: he lost because he got old. The same is true whether the bodybuilder is a bodybuilding champion or not. Nobody brought up the fact that he did not train hard, was out of shape, or no longer had the will and ambition to succeed.

A non-competitive bodybuilder's issue is that as he ages, his obligations increase. He marries, has children, needs to work to support a family, and frequently attends school to advance. He needs to find time for parents' night, help with schoolwork, and pick up the kids from school. His wife also wants him to make time for family activities.

With everything going on, it's easy to skip a day or two at the gym, and before you know it, you're working out less and less. Eventually, one day you wake up unfit, overweight, and slow. You become aware that it has been a while since you last trained.

As I close the door to my room at bedtime, I find myself looking up at the ceiling. I tried to workout today and things did not go as expected. Is it time to quit working out for good? Am I too old? When will I know when to quit exercising? Will I be ready to leave what I loved so much all of my life?

No, not us. We will continue to train as long as God permits. When I'm working out at the gym, I hear those voices from far away. I have crossed into another word. I tell myself, one more set, one more rep. I have been here before and I know about it. I have a theory about speed and endurance in my own special way. I think I've found what keeps me young both intellectually and physically.

More than 50 years ago, I found out the hard way that champions are born, and that I did not have the good genes from my parents to get big and strong. Trying to get there, I sustained injuries; tennis elbows, infringement shoulders, you name it. At 5'9 ½", my top weight only got to 185 pounds, but somehow I felt slow and sluggish. I realized that when I practiced my other activities, such as boxing and martial arts, I was slow and easily exhausted. I discovered that at a weight of 175 pounds, I felt strong and agile, I could hit and move. I don't have a bodybuilder's body; I don't look like one, but I'm one and I train very much like one.

I discovered that I had been doing more than was necessary. I had to put in an hour or more four or five days a week. Exercises are frequently so demanding that many people get injuries.

I've maintained the same weight since high school and barely a two-inch increase in waist size. I reside in Miami, not far from a stunning, sizable park. My occasional training location is here. A few years ago, I occasionally competed with younger guys my age. I discovered that I could outperform them in activities such as running 1/8 mile, doing push-ups, and boxing a round or two. Sometimes we raced up the stairs to two or three floors, and when we reached the top.

I just walked for a short time, breathing deeply a few times, and I was recovered. I was able to talk easily while the other guys had to hold themselves to the rail, wall, or place their hands on their knees and gasp for air for quite a few minutes.

I'm not young anymore, but I can run almost as fast as I did in high school. I can lift more weight than I ever have in my life. Am I too old? I don't care if I don't weigh 200 pounds or if I have a 19-inch arm or not.

This episode made me think it might be an interesting magazine article. My training can make you look younger, feel better, and probably live longer.

I have learned in my years of working out that exercising is the fountain of youth; exercise is crucial for having a sharp, active, and appealing body.

The common signs of aging are infirmity, frailty, loss of energy, your height diminishes, and you replace fat where there was muscle. Chronological age is unavoidable, but physiological age is not. You can have the outward appearance and internal system of someone fifty years old or thirty-five years old. Looking great is desirable.

The first thing I do is I never ever pick a book whose title mentions anything about age or aging. What for? I still do most of the exercises I did in high school. I can still kick higher than my head, like I used to.

I keep my mind sharp by reading all kinds of books; somehow I get along better with younger people, at parties, anywhere, probably because of my 30 years as a professor. I know that all this kept me young in body and mind. I'm convinced that talking with younger people will keep you young. The conversation is a much younger one. Older people tend to talk about sickness or injuries, and somehow it affects their wellbeing too.

There's no better anti-aging strategy in the world than daily exercise. In some studies, it's been found that it strengthens bones, keeps muscles toned, improves flexibility, increases circulation, lowers blood pressure, improves blood sugar control, and keeps oxygen flowing to the brain, heart, and lungs. And according to new research, regular exercise cannot only increase the ability of the brain to function, but it can actually increase its size. One of the main reasons I train my body is so that my mind works effectively.

The best anti-aging exercise program incorporates both cardiovascular and weight training to keep your muscles strong, toned, and youthful; helps control your weight; and keeps your metabolic rate humming.

Exercising, taking walks, reading, socializing with family and friends, drinking red wine, not smoking, eating wisely will keep young.

Most of the bodybuilding books/magazines are written, I believe, and lose their target. Most training programs are designed for athletes or champions, leaving the average person in limbo.

What this regular person wants is a more youthful appearance, strength, stamina, an increase in muscle mass, a reduction of excess body fat, tone, a more attractive abdomen, and an improvement in respiratory endurance. Not to mention conditioning of the heart, it has been recorded that exercise improves physical efficiency, reduces cardiac stress, lowers the systolic and diastolic pressure, and lowers blood lipids, especially triglycerides.

The image of a champion bodybuilder these days is of veins about to pop, many times gasping for air, and some have a belly that looks pregnant. In the old days, you had symmetrical appearances and small waistlines, making the body attractive and pleasant to look at. People like Steve Reeves, Dave Draper, Frank Zane, and Sergio Oliva, to mention a few.

My training consists of Bodyweight Blasts variations, a program similar to Cross Fit training but not a specific fitness program. I never do the same exercises twice. I learn by doing this that I keep injuries away. I do heavy weight training (heavy for me) today, rest the next day, and then I do mix-cardio, jumping Jacks, stationary running, rope jumping, or spring-walks in the park, and shadowboxing at the same time.

I also walk on a one-foot high, four-inch wide concrete edging, closing my eyes for a few feet, alternating slow or fast walks with open or closed eyes. I do this for balance. This requires core stability and a lot of practice.

I alternate the exercises every week and the sequence. I rest a day, then do light weight exercises. Sometimes I train for two consecutive days, then rest for two. I also keep the workout short, never more than 40 minutes. I move from one exercise to the other as fast as I can, resting just enough to get back my breath. If I'm tired, I take an extra day in between exercises. What I look forward to is cardiovascular and respiratory endurance, strength, flexibility, power, speed, coordination, agility, and balance.

You may never be a top bodybuilder champion, but you will develop a great body. You bet this program can build muscles, especially for the trainee who hasn't changed his program for a long time and has hit a plateau. For me, it works great!

I liked to mix up my workouts and avoided repeating the same exercise or workout order. I like mixing up routines, exercises, sets, reps, rest times, and workout orders, never allowing the muscles to get used to the stress I'm placing on them. This is how I do it.

If I did three exercises for the chest in one workout, on the next chest workout I would do three completely different exercises for the chest. And so on.

I think the weight of an athlete should not matter; it is how he looks or feels. If he looks and feels great, then he is great. When a bodybuilder or athlete is just too heavy just for the sake of being big, then his physique and health suffer.

You should always warm up and cool down. My warm up is simple; I move a little around, and if I'm doing weight training, I do my first exercise with a very light weight and then go up in weight. If doing cardio, just move around a little first to get the blood moving and get the heart and lungs ready. At first, go easy. For the cool down, I do a couple of stretching exercises for supple muscles, especially for the legs, arms, and neck. I do this kind of training on an empty stomach, just water and coffee.

The effect I get from this is amazing, and my fat ratio has been amazing. I know some experts believe otherwise, but in my case, it works perfectly. You have to get used to it, but once you're used to it, it's great. Then, you have what I call breakfast-lunch and feel strong for the rest of the day.

You don't have to eliminate foods or beverages. What matters is portion size and food quality. Don't eat like this is the last meal you are going to have. This is the trick. The concept of the wide variety and portions would pay off.

I eat everything I want. I just leave a little food on the plate. Sometimes I split a big dinner plate with my wife. I don't drink soda; instead, I drink water; I drink three or four beer bottles per week and maybe a half-bottle of wine per week; and my cholesterol and blood pressure have never been better.

You don't have to spend a penny to try my system. There are no gimmicks to buy or pills to swallow. Except for your regular barbell and dumbbells, your regular gym, and your body, no special equipment is required.

Some bodybuilders in the gym were not progressing; they had hit a plateau. A few tried my routine for two months and were impressed with the change. Less fat, more cuts, better symmetry, tone, the upper body, calves, and the legs took on a more muscular look. Even the way they walk and stand is much more impressive. I advised them to return to their regular routine after two months and to try it again a few months later.

A flat belly looks great. However, it takes a tremendous amount of effort. You don't really need one as hard as a rock. You can have a pleasing abdomen with a trim of fat that looks good in clothes as well as in a swim trunk. If you don't feel good about yourself, you are sending ineffective signals to another person. These signals are sex appeal.

An intense burst of activity in a short time can give you complete and fast results. You can achieve more progress in 30 minutes of interval training done three or four times a week than people training an hour or more five days a week. Why not try smarter, follow my combination workouts, and see what it can do for you?

You will all lose weight around your waist; your figure will improve, you will exchange flab for solid lean muscle mass, and your muscular strength and respiratory endurance will improve. You will discover the fountain of youth.

Inactivity will kill you.

What to expect:
Improved muscle definition and gain lean muscle mass.
Lower BMI (body mass index).
Increase in strength and energy.
It reduces recovery time.
Better-quality sleep.

I'm thrilled to be able to maintain a very high level of fitness at my age by adhering to a program like the one I've laid out for you.

The magazine is no longer available in print.

Like father like son

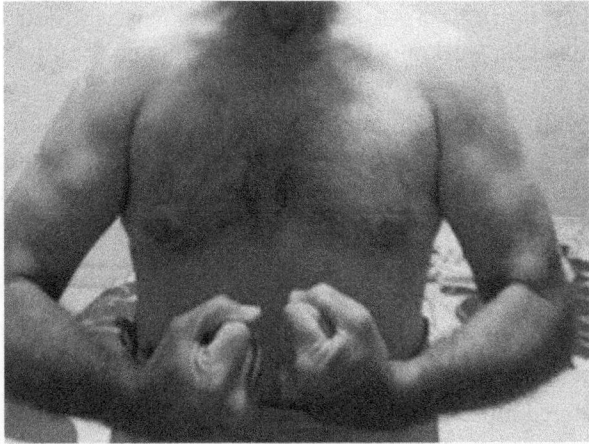

The author continues to exercise after 50 years of training.

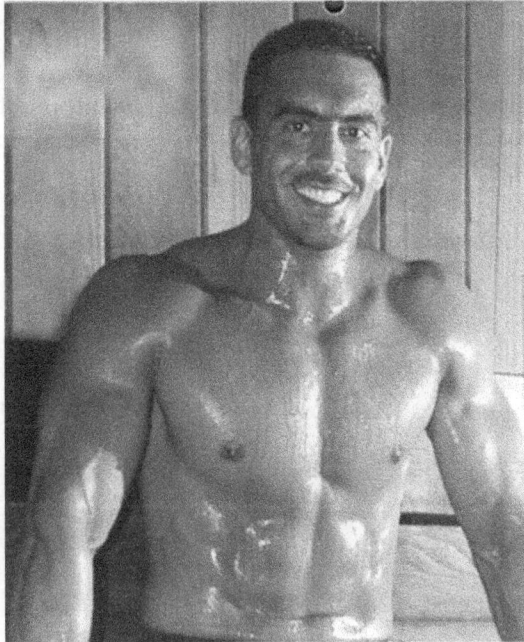

Frank Marchante Jr.

The Mature Weight Gainer

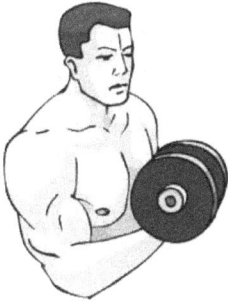

Don't force yourself to eat. Eat small portions three or four times a day. Don't over train or train for too long. Do heavy, short workouts, but don't use super heavy weights. Use lighter weights and do more reps. Have one bowel movement a day. Eat well-balanced foods and plenty of protein.

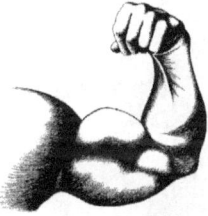

You may add one or two protein shakes with a multi-vitamin and mineral pill a day. To gain size, let's say you are doing bench presses with a 150-lb. 12 to 18 reps. You will not gain size like that. If you add 20 or 30 pounds and do 6 to 8 reps, you will gain size. Keep adding weight. This is the way to put on size. Eat whatever you can or want, keep track of junk food, and train 4 or 5 times a week. Stay with basic exercises like squats, rows, curls and so on. Limit your cardiovascular activity a little. Working only your large muscles, relaxing, and enjoying life are the keys to success.

The Mature Weight Reducer

Reduce the number of food portions in your meals; eat a variety of healthy, high-quality foods. Eat a lot of fruits and vegetables. Eliminate junk foods like cakes, desserts, sodas, candy, etc. Don't eat late in the evening. Have one bowel movement a day. Leave food on your plate. Share food when eating out.

Do cardiovascular exercises like walking or cycling three or four times a week for at least half an hour. Don't diet; develop a long-term healthy nutrition plan. Take your time getting there; you didn't get fat overnight.

Aspirin - The Wonder Drug

1 -Anti- inflammatory properties
2- Anti-pyretic lower fever
3- Analgesic-relieves pain
4- Blocks formation of platelets in blood vessels
5- Reduces the risk of heart attacks and strokes

Some people take enteric aspirin for the long haul. People take one daily or one every two days. In some people aspirin increases the risk of internal bleeding. Check with your doctor first for advice on this wonder drug.

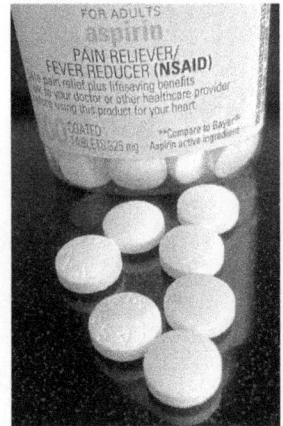

Exercise

The Super Tranquilizer:
Evidence shows that exercising can help you in many ways. Check the following list:

1. More energy, better health
2. Stronger muscles, tendons, and ligaments
3. Clears thoughts and mind
4. Able to concentrate more
5. Improve your memory
6. Better self-confidence
7. A sense of physical well-being
8. Helps you sleep better, sooner, deeper
9. Fights depression and pain
10. 100% better body image

Steroids

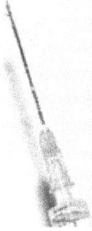

Steroids have been around for a long time. Doctor John Ziegler, together with the Ciba lab, produced Dianabol in 1956. Later, other steroids such as Deca, Winstrol, and Anavar were developed.

Common names among users are words like stacking, staggering, descending doses, ascending doses, tapering, and shot gunning, among others. A popular stack among many others is Testosterone, Insulin, and GH. In my opinion, what some bodybuilders are doing is crazy. Some champions are injecting steroids, drugs, and GH into their bodies. This is crazy, very crazy.

Some popular steroids are:

Anavar	Androl
Maxibolon	Stromba
Winstrol V	Testosterone
Deca-durabolin	Turinabol
Primobolon	Equipoise
Dianabol	Masteron

Common Street names for steroids

Gym Candy	Juice
Roids	Gear
Arnolds	Stackers
Weight Trainers	

Alzheimer's disease

A recent study conducted by researchers from the neurology department at Columbia University Medical Center in New York has observed the possible effects of the standard diet eaten by people in countries around the Mediterranean Sea, such as Greece. The "Mediterranean diet" consists of mostly fruits, vegetables, and beans, as well as fish, olive oil, a reasonable amount of wine, selected dairy foods, and small amounts of meat and chicken.

However, more studies are needed to confirm these results. However, the results indicate a reduced risk of developing Alzheimer's and a lower mortality rate among those who contracted the disease.

Randolph Schiffer, MD, is director of the Cleveland Clinic Lou Ruvo Center for Brain Health in Cleveland. With that said, most of us in the Alzheimer's research field believe that people should adopt and continue healthy lifestyles, including diets low in saturated fats and high in antioxidants and B vitamins.

Olive Oil:

Researchers have become interested in the anti-inflammatory benefits of olive oil because people who eat a traditional Mediterranean diet (which is rich in olive oil) seem to have fewer health conditions related to inflammation, such as degenerative joint diseases or diabetes.

Olive Oil Can Reduce the Risk of Alzheimer's Disease

Numerous studies, including one recently published in the journal Chemical Neuroscience, showed that the Oleocanthal in extra virgin olive oil has the potential to reduce the risk of Alzheimer's disease and the cognitive decline that comes with aging.

Italian academics from the University of Florence have found that extra virgin olive oil polyphenols may prevent or slow down the appearance of Alzheimer's disease.

Olive oil polyphenols are known to be powerful antioxidants that may help to reverse oxidative damage that occurs in the aging process.

The researchers concluded that their results support the possibility that dietary supplementation with extra virgin olive oil may prevent or delay the occurrence of Alzheimer's disease and reduce the severity of its symptoms.

The Olive Oil Diet Lowers the Risk of Type 2 Diabetes

A study published in the scientific journal Diabetes Care showed that a Mediterranean-style diet rich in olive oil reduced the risk of type II diabetes by almost 50 percent compared to a low-fat diet. Type II diabetes is the most common and preventable form of diabetes. Be careful because of the caloric content and fat, which put you at risk of weight gain, high and blood pressure.

Fake oil

Be careful with fake olive oil.
One step to increasing your chances of buying real olive oil that is actually what it says it is: turn the bottle over and read the back label.

You'll see an expiration date (usually two years after an oil has been bottled), but what you're looking for in particular is the harvest date; the further away the two-year date is, the fresher the oil is.

Prepare yourself. Real olive oil is strong and it will catch in your throat. You are going to cough. Your eyes may water. These are symptoms that what you taste is authentic.

Common training injuries

Runners' Knees: You can touch the swelling under the kneecap, and it hurts, especially when you walk.

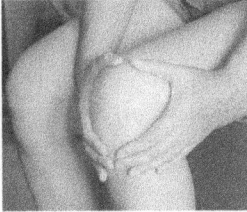

Tennis elbow-It hurts and you feel pain inside, outside, or back of your forearm very close to your elbows. This is the famous tennis elbow.

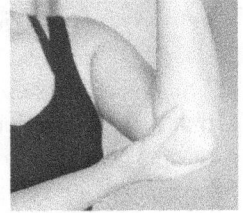

Strain- In many cases, the strain is mild and is just overstretching of the muscle with no evident tear. The result could be pain and discomfort with motion.

Rice means **rest, ice, compression** and **elevation**

Treatment
The first thing to do with sports injuries is what is known as RICE. For a very long time, doctors had a lot of disagreements about when or if you should apply ice. Many doctors are telling you to apply ice today. There is a famous orthopedic surgeon near where I live in Miami, FL, who is completely against using ice; he says you may develop arthritis by using ice on an injury. When you visit any therapy office in Miami, Florida, they immediately won't use ice if this experienced specialist doctor gave you a therapy referral.

There are numerous over-the-counter remedies you can buy to reduce your pain and inflammation, like Ibuprofen, Alive, and, of course, Aspirin, the king of over-the-counter pain relievers.

If you get injured or experience some kind of pain or discomfort, take a few days off, take a pain reliever, and relax for a couple of days. If the pain persists, make an appointment with your doctor or an orthopedic doctor. He will probably probably inject you with some cortisone, and you will recover soon after the injection.

Conclusion

In closing I'm pleased to have gotten a very nice level of fitness following the course I've given you. This book won't make you a Mr. Universe or Ms. Universe, but if you follow the advice, you will develop an envy-worthy body and incredible shape.

So there you have it: all the methods necessary to develop a kick-ass training program that will help you shed body fat like never before!

To say that I know all the answers would be a lie. Like I said thru the book there is no one size fits all approach to obtain a trim, muscular, healthy body.

You have taken the time to read this book. It is now time to start doing the workouts in this book and follow the instructions. This is the last page of this book, but my goal is for you to put the advice given here to work for the rest of your life. You won't regret it.

This book is not the final word for either men or women, but it is the beginning of a commitment to developing a lean, sensual, attractive, muscular figure if you choose to spend time to working out and caring for your body.

Now let's put this book down, get ready, and start working out.

Muscle up databases are a perfectly clear, instructional and motivational read for...the man or woman, athlete, home trainer, gym trainer, and even the professional personal trainer."

Denie

Terminologies worth knowing

Aerobics
Activity that relies on the intake of oxygen for energy.

Abs
Term for abdominal muscle or midsection.

Interval training-HIT
Short, fast work alternated with slow work.

Absorption
The process in which nutrients are passed into the bloodstream.

The Amino acids
Building blocks of protein molecules are necessary for every bodily process.

Anabolic Steroids (Steroids)
A drug taken from a male hormone (testosterone) or prepared synthetically, to aid body growth.

Antioxidant
A chemical molecule that prevents oxygen from reacting with other compounds and protects cells from damage.

Aspirin
The chemical name Acetylsalicylic acid reduces inflammation and fever.

Barbells
A basic steel bar affixed with plates on both ends.

Bodybuilding
Activity to achieve body perfection

Bulk up
Gaining muscle mass

Calorie
The way in which energy is measured from food

Cardio
Aerobic activity is defined as exercise good for the heart and lungs.

Carbohydrates
Sugar and starches in food.

The Cardiovascular System
The heart, together with arteries and veins, transports nutrients and oxygen to tissues and organs.

Cheating
Body motion to help with an exercise

Cortisol
A catabolic hormone contributes to fat storage, a product of stress.

Cholesterol
A fat substance found in the brain and blood in excess would give you arteriosclerosis and heart disease.

D.H.E.A
Steroids secreted naturally by the adrenal glands.

Definition
Muscularity with less fat covering the muscles.

Dumbbells
Short steel with affixed weight plates.

FDA
The FDA is the Food and Drug Administration.

Glutes maximus
Glutes, butts, and rear muscles found in the human buttocks.

Glucose
Blood sugar is a major source of energy in humans. It circulates in the bloodstream.

Hormonal
We have about 50 different kinds of hormones. Greek words.

Human Growth Hormone
The hormone secreted by the pituitary gland regulates growth and is released, especially during sleep.

Insulin
Hormones secreted by the pancreas transport blood sugar into cells for energy.

Isometric exercise
They don't require you to move or bend any joints.

Isotonic exercises
This involves straining the muscles while moving the joints and applying force.

EZ-curl
Bent barbell to protect your wrists and elbows.

Jogging and running
It is excellent for cardiovascular health, bone density.

Body tissues made of fibers are able to contract in response to the nervous system.

Metabolism
Scientists use it to describe the chemical processes in the body, especially the use that involves nutrients.

Sprints
Intensity is moving very fast as you can maintain for a designated time (10 to 40 seconds) or short marked distance followed by a recovery pace during interval training.

Somatotrapin
Another name for human growth hormone.

Plyometric exercises
Is a type of training that uses the speed and force of various movements to build muscle and power.

Pineal Gland
Is a small, pea-shaped gland located in the brain that produces melatonin. Melatonin influences sexual development and moderate sleep.

Pituitary Gland
A small gland at the base of the brain. It produces hormones that regulate growth and sexual development, and it shrinks as we age.

Proteins
Group of organic nitrogen compounds. The main building materials for muscles, blood, skin, hair, and organs. The word protein means "most important." Hippocrates named it 2500 years ago.

Testosterone
In men, this is the primary sex hormone.

Repetition
One single movement

Vitamins
It is required by the body for growth, development, and cell repair.

Isotonic exercises
Straining the muscles while moving the joints and applying force.

Isometric exercises
They don't require you to move or to bend any joints.

About the Author

Frank Marchante was a Florida educator, a Pear teacher, and head of Department for 30 years. He is retired now. In 2000, he was one of the 30 professors selected in North America to participate in the People to People Ambassador Program in the Delegation of Counselors and Technology Education to the Republic of China. His selection was based on his professional experience, credentials, and competency.

Marchante, a huge fan of the sport of bodybuilding, became involved in bodybuilding in the Golden Era. Through his life, he has trained many young men in bodybuilding including his own son Frank Jr. who won 2nd place in a 2002 bodybuilding contest in Miami. He has owned a home personal gym for the last 50 years.

With his advice, he has aided many women and men in their quest for a slimmer, stronger, and healthier body with his guidance, instruction, and training techniques. Resistance and callisthenic training have been introduced by the author to encourage and motivate teenagers, men, women, and even the elderly. Through personal experience in the classroom, he trained teenagers to be admitted to football teams and females to swim teams.

He was the speaker and recipient of the "Hall of Fame" Award for Mr. Olympia Sergio Oliva in February 2004 in Florida and the speaker who introduced champion Sergio Oliva at a South Florida Bodybuilding Championship in 2004.

He started learning karate when he was 12 years old and afterwards transitioned to studying Wing Chun kun-Fu training for many years. At the same time, his father started teaching him how to box.

Frank has taken part in numerous adventures, including ascents to one of Bolivia's highest peaks, Illimani, at 20,742 feet high, one of the highest mountain peaks in the Andes, and the eighteenth highest peak in South America, all while wearing an oxygen mask and walking through the clouds, with snow up to his knees.

He ventured deep by foot into the deep, dark, and dense, dangerous, and inevitably Amazon jungles in Bolivia and Peru. Drove through The World's Most Dangerous Road in Bolivia—The Death Road in 1971.

He traveled across the intimidating Titicaca Lake, the highest lake in the world, in an Indian canoe accompanied by an Indian from Bolivia to Peru 50 years ago, before tourists began visiting the lake.

He climbed the massive volcano of Popocatepetl, Mexico, the second highest in Mexico and North America's second highest volcano at 5,452 meters (17,887 feet) above sea level. He has also hang–glided from a very high peak in Acapulco city and has also done parasailing in Acapulco and Cozumel.

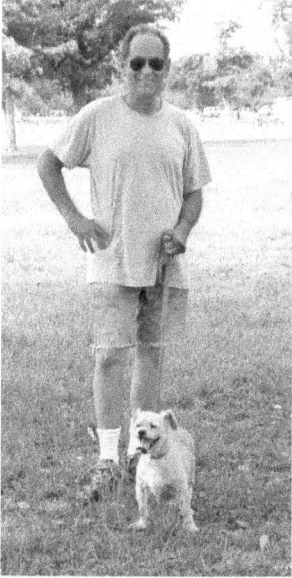

The Author AM running-walks with his dog Tobby

He took his first flying lessons in the early 70s at Tamiami airport in South Miami in a Piper Cherokee 140, where at the end of the 80s he kept his own plane, a Panther 2+.

He applied in 1986 to NASA when the teacher educator space program was going into space in the shuttle Challenger, but he was not chosen. The shuttle exploded 73 seconds after liftoff.

He has written articles for newspapers and magazines. He is the author of published books like Sergio Oliva the Myth, El Atentado del Siglo (The Ultimate Target), Streetwise Extreme-Surviving the Unexpected, there are many pages in the internet from Russia to France discussing his books.

His other passions are sport flying, composing music, reading, and traveling.

Photo Credit:

The author has made every effort to identify the source of all photos reproduced in this book. Every effort has been made to trace the ownership of each photograph and to provide full acknowledgement for its use. "No copyright infringement is intended"

If any errors have occurred, they will be corrected in subsequent editions, provided notification is sent to the publisher. (Several photos that appear in this book have no identification of the photographer who took them or the subject model.) We regret that the photographer could not be credited in the proper way.

Additional photos courtesy of:
Frank Marchante--- Denie

Freepick.com "Designed by Freepik"
Drobotdean men double bicep back pose shoulder& Girl abdomen black cut up shirt, Lyashenko girl sideway holding two dumbbells, Sergeycau chest pose sideway & seating concentrated curl, Jcompx men-girl hands on waist & couple stretching arms up, Serhii-bo men 3 photos using cables-bands, Drobotdean woman doing bench press with bands, Lyashenko girls front holding two dumbbells, Pressfotox men jumping rope, Valuavitalyx girl butt from back sideways hands on behind, Master1305 girl holding jump rope sideway, Standret Couple lunges, Pressphotox men holding rope, Racool-St close up Men barbell curl, Master103Men strong facing front.

Pixabay.com
Fabricio Macedo back bikini girl getting into the ocean with surfboard, Klimkin girl shadowboxing, Luxstorm girl right side holding two dumbbells, Dejavupics81 girl laying in sand pretty face, Pixabay men hitting bag, Xusenru girl posterior beach, Andreaaltini sexy girl drinking water, Deedee86 girl measuring tape waist, No name girl doing knees raises in floor, Sapper-designs girl lat pulley behind neck, DanEvans pregnant woman at beach, Asad Malvides girl holding tennis elbows, Nattanan23 girl holding knees pain, Pixabay Fitness Dumbell sign & bodybuilding black silhouette, Harutmovsisyan men wrapping hands.

Freeimages.com
Yorgos03 back shoulder arm extended
Harutmovsisyan girl beach white bikini sideway

Pexels.com
Anete Lusina barbell plate, Andrea Piacquadio free men squats & bike
girl, Daniel Torobekov front bikini girl walking, Anush Gorak men front
barbell black background curl, Anush Gorak men torso side way
abdomen, Nathan Cowley lady cutting food, Oscar Machado reverse
hands barbell rows, João Jesus woman coming out pool with hat, by
Panther black men back & chest, Pexel element Element5 woman legs
riding stationary bike, Li sun men doing burpies, Pexel photo hands
holding medicine ball, TiaMiroshnichenko girl back with boxing gloves
& girl jumping rope no shoes, Jonathan Borba girl doing cardio in eclipse
machine, Asad Maldives bikini girl back beach, Karolin Grabowska girl
front dumbbell front raises, Omer Karakus men torso right sideway-
abdomen, Zaid Ali men chest sideway, Lyashenko Girl in sand reading
book, Behrouz Sasani men torso hands on waist, Sahil Khaliq men across
arm chest & men arms across chest holding wrist, Woman legs crossed
cottonbro, Woman legs againt bench Marta Wave, Airam Dato Woman
cut up shirt front jeans, Polina Tankilevitch girl doing lunges, Nappy girl
stair, Elena Shekhovtcova girls legs up facing down.

Unplash.com
Igor Starkov surfboard girl standing front, Abby Savage wood cutting,
Dorothea Oldani Cuban girl running, Erick Miclean men side close up
dumbbell curls, Sfanfu Gheorghe washing car, Andres Gomez girl back
bend beach gymnastic & dumbbell racks, Dario Luna Marquez girl
gyrating back in beach, Federico-Faccipieri girl-boy throwing medicine
ball wall, Liam Johnson front men black t-shirt barbell curl, Carlos-
Augusto-close up girl back with surfboard, Damir-spanic close-up men
dumbbell right arm with veins with black t-shirt, Tyler-nix girl going up
stairs sideway, Houcine Ncib black-girl stretching arm overhead bikini,
Pipe Gil girl standing in beach by umbrella, Scott-webb girl doing leg
press ride side view, Huba Inc girl measuring waist black bikini.

Dreamstime

Udoudo (girl: Waist measuring girl almost sideway

Note: After intense and long hours, we regret that we could not find the name of the model or the photographer who took the picture of an attractive girl sideways with a trim waist in jeans, to credit.

Mike Mentzer and Dave Draper courtesy of GMV Productions LTD Wayne Gallasch.

Additional resources:

In researching for this book I relied on numerous sources in the writing of this book. Publications and websites proved valuable throughout the entire process. Although the list is not exhaustive, some of them are included:

Media related -Periodicals books

Building the Ultimate Physique-Sergio Oliva and Frank Marchante

Classic Anatomy Bodybuilding-Steve Speyrer

Brother Iron Sister Steel –Dave Draper

Heart of Steel-Dan Lurie and David Robson

Beef It-Robert Kennedy

Raw Muscle! Robert Kennedy and Dennis Weis

Rock Hard Abs-Robert Kennedy

Unleashing The Wild Physique-Vince Gironda and Robert Kennedy

Mass! Robert Kennedy and Dennis Weis

Magazines:

Flex

Health and Strength

Iron Man

La Culture Physique

Mr. America

Muscle and Fitness

Muscle Builder

Musclemag International

Muscle Training Illustrated

Muscle Development

Planet Muscle

Reps

Periodicals / websites

https://www.classicanatomygym.net

https://gmvbodybuilding.com -Bodybuilding Videos

https://www.davedraper.com

https://www.labrada.com

https://aniballopez.com/

http://www.caseyviator.com/

Mayo Clinic -- https://www.mayoclinic.org/

Academy of General Dentistry- https: //agd.org/

Centers for Disease Control and Prevention- https://www.cdc.gov/

The American Academy of Dermatology- https://www.aad.org/

Medical and health information https://www.medicalnewstoday.com/

Health news- https://www.webmd.com/

American Cancer Society https://www.cancer.org/

Florida Heart Association   https://www.heart.org/en/affiliates/Florida

ALS Disease Association   https://www.als.org/

American Lung Association   https://www.lung.org/

American Diabetes Association https://www.diabetes.org/

Miami Lighthouse/Blind Visually Impaired https://miamilighthouse.org/

Reviews

The author, Frank Marchante, has provided a one-stop for all the tools you need to acquire a healthy, trim, and sexy body for both men and women.

Tony Bart

Marchante has done a terrific job creating a routine that any woman or man can follow. I highly recommend it.

Personal trainer Jim Okant

If you want a book to obtain a remarkable body, no matter if you are a woman, a man, or over 50, this is it. This book is for you.

Christina Lopez

If you use the techniques in this book, your friends will be astounded.

Gym's owner Ab Haoei

This is the first book I ever recommended to obtain a strong, new-trimmed, and incredible body.

Supervisor fitness supplements Albert Minett

This book is worth the purchase price. An encyclopedia of complete information on obtaining an amazing body.

Harriet Naji

This book has really spiced up not only my cardio workouts but the breakdown of each workout to keep me motivated and focused.

Denise Limpton Fitness spokesperson

This is a handy, concise, and informative book, by far the best book of its kind, full of photographs.

Olive Piapot

Gras Publishing Present

Sergio Oliva the Myth

Sergio Oliva, The Myth, the only man to have ever won the Mr. Olympia title uncontested. Now at last Oliva tells all. His early childhood, his daring escape from a communist country to gain his freedom, and how he developed his once in a lifetime, out of this world, Herculean and powerful body with perfect symmetry and mind blowing proportions that made him the most muscular and incredible body of all time. Learn the facts behind the world's most prestigious and famous contests.

Sergio Oliva

THE MYTH
His Life Story
and....

Complete
Guide to:

Explosive
Growth

Mr. Olympia
Mr. World
Mr.Universe

Collossal
Muscle Mass

Awesome
Strength

Ultra Ripped
Muscularity

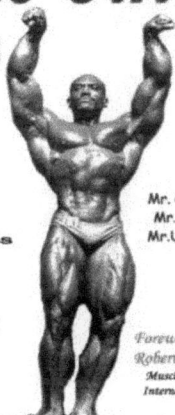

Foreword By:
Robert Kennedy
MuscleMag
International

Building The Ultimate Physique
With Frank Marchante

Get a front row seat as Sergio describes his confrontations with Arnold Schwarzenegger. Nothing is held back as Sergio speaks his mind.

Sergio discusses Bodybuilding Politics, Drugs and more. Find thrilling action and suspense, unlike any other bodybuilder's book.

And
• Maximum Muscle Development • A Seminar with Sergio-Over 100 Q & A's • Sergio Oliva's Training Secret Routines • Steroids-GH, Interaction of Growth Hormone • Get in Shape Routines for Women • The Myth's Health Recipes.
And much more!

"Sergio Oliva is to bodybuilding what Babe Ruth is to baseball."
  Lee Labrada –Champion

"A complete package of mass, symmetry, and definition!"
  Jay Cutler – Mr. Olympia

Notes

www.ingramcontent.com/pod-product-compliance
Lightning Source LLC
Chambersburg PA
CBHW020604270326
41927CB00005B/164